Describing Care

Describing Care

Image and Practice
in Rehabilitation

Jaber F. Gubrium
David R. Buckholdt

Marquette University

 Oelgeschlager, Gunn & Hain, Publishers, Inc.
Cambridge, Massachusetts

International Standard Book Number: 0-89946-135-2

Library of Congress Catalog Card Number: 81-18774

Printed in West Germany

Library of Congress Cataloging in Publication Data

Gubrium, Jaber F.
  Describing care.

  Bibliography: p.
  Includes index.
  1. Rehabilitation. I. Buckholdt, David R.
II. Title. [DNLM: 1. Rehabilitation—Organization and administration. 2. Data collection—Methods. WB 320 G92ld]
RM930.G8   362.4   81-18774
ISBN 0-89946-135-2   AACR2

*For Suzanne
and Shelley*

Contents

Preface

This book is one outgrowth of an ongoing research project, the general focus of which is the social organization of care in human service institutions. The theme of the research is that the character of problems serviced—from emotional disturbance to paraplegia, stroke, and senility—is as much a product of caretakers' practices as it is a feature of the behavior and lives of those cared for. Here, we examine physical rehabilitation as it is organized and practiced in a rehabilitation hospital by physical therapists, occupational therapists, speech therapists, social workers, leisure therapists, nurses, and physicians.

Our interpretation of the data is based on a simple premise: what is known about things is significantly related to how things are described and the conditions of description. While commonplace, this tenet is rarely the explicit focus of research. In portraying the therapies, treatments, and deliberations of clinical staff, we attempt to show—to display for the reader—how staff members work up descriptions of activities from particular conditions, using their knowledge of audience relevance in organizing what they say and write. We refer to the working up as "practice" and to the knowledge of audience relevance as "image." Accordingly, we find that what is to be heard or read by select audiences (patients, families, other professionals, insurance companies) about physical rehabilitation is not just a better or worse description of rehabilitation activity but an audience-specific, staff-articulated description of it.

We are concerned with two implications of the theme and data: what the research implies about description in general and what it suggests about the character of human service accountability in particular. Because all description is, at some time or other, a human activity, it is subject to the everyday practical conditions of that activity. To evaluate a description, in principle, as reliable and valid is to gloss over the practice of describing, something that is a cardinal feature of much evaluation research and social research methodology. Description cannot be separated from its practice. When we center attention on the descriptions offered by people who are formally charged with responsibility for accurately depicting professional activity, the general implication applies in particular. Because accountability is subject to beliefs about audience relevance and expectations, to be accountable means to be able to produce adequate accounts, which—together with concerns over accuracy—complicates the matter of accountability far beyond how it is currently understood.

Our method was to observe and interact with the clinical staff of a hospital as they went about their work and described it. Some of the work and description was therapeutic, in which case we assisted therapists in activities like power-building, range-of-motion evaluation, and test administration. Some was informative, which was observed in staff's casual encounters with families and significant others as well as in more formal conferences. Some description justified payment for services rendered. This we also observed in what were called "team conferences" or "utilization reviews." Always carrying a theme, the method aimed to reveal the practice of description within the purview of staff understandings of rehabilitation and how to present it.

Images and practice are pervasive features of social life in that, however people behave, they act against a background of select understandings of their actions and articulate them in relation to specific everyday affairs. Yet some social settings seem to make image and practice highly visible, places where people have a wide range of expectations about normal activities. The physical rehabilitation hospital is such a place, where there is a staff whose conception of the meaning of rehabilitation ranges from medical to educational and custodial understandings, a staff who in turn is accountable to audiences with the same range of understandings. It is a more poignant setting in this regard than an acute care hospital, where care expectations are commonly articulated in terms of medicine, or a school, where for the most part learning, not curing, is the central image. The rehabilitation hospital, more than many human service settings, brings image and practice to our attention as a routine feature of its normal activities.

Chapter 1, "The Process of Clinical Description," begins with a discussion of the central place of description in everyday life and continues by introducing key concepts such as "descriptive circumstance," "descriptive goodness," and "descriptive adequacy." The participants and clinical routine of a physical rehabilitation hospital are briefly presented, the hospital being a setting where much activity is devoted to describing care. Chapter 2, "Images and the Descriptive Process," considers in detail the diverse images that enter into the hospital's descriptive activity.

Chapters 3, 4, and 5 are substantive, documenting by means of gestural and conversational data how three different staff audiences serve to organize the images of rehabilitation presented to them by staff members. Respectively, the data are interpreted to show how the working patient, families, and third parties (such as insurance companies) are told "different" yet truthful and specific things about clinical activities and patient progress.

Chapter 6, "Accountability," takes up the implications of descriptive practice for the vision of accuracy common to many models of accountability. It ends with a section on "accounting practice," in which formal accountability itself is brought full-circle to image and practice.

Acknowledgments

We are indebted to Marquette University for the many ways in which it served to underwrite the research reported in the book. John Oh, Dean of the Graduate School, provided funds for the preparation of the manuscript. Irene Cunningham, Shirley Frick, and Linda Hall typed it.

The project was facilitated by the Wilshire Hospital staff. We are grateful to Wilshire's administrator for his concern and encouragement, the therapists for their patience and help in gaining an understanding of clinical routine and descriptive practice, the patients for their openness and good humor, and the families for their efforts on our behalf.

Several graduate students responded to and constructively criticized our working ideas and interpretations of data: Virginia Bowen, Cheryl Carpenter, Joan Dinan, Peggy Dunn, Robert Lynott, and Sharon O'Gorman. Their enthusiasm and insight are much appreciated.

Thanks to Joyce Olesen for her fine copyediting.

Chapter 1

The Process of Clinical Description

Much of everyday activity involves describing, informing, or reporting. We may be asked "What's new?" or "What's happening?" and respond with information or descriptions that serve as the working stuff of casual conversation. Or in our professions we may be required to complete formal reports that describe activities or events that are our special responsibilities. Our descriptions, however, are not limited to depictions of fact; they also comprise ideas, sentiments, and opinions. Whether the setting is casual or formal, whether the topic is abstract or specific, description presents a spoken or written message about something.

In some sense, we all know that descriptions are not actually the conditions, events, or individuals described. We have all wondered whether what we are being told is true, accurate—whether we are hearing someone "tell it like it is," or whether the information is being filtered mainly for the audience's benefit. Thus when we describe something, we decide not only what information to present but also how to present it for the desired effect.

We know that while we may be focusing on particular situations or problems we also come to recognize them by hearing or reading descriptions. When descriptions are presented to us by others, we know things through their reports. When we look at something and describe it to ourselves or to others, we may wonder whether our eyes are really seeing what we think they are. The degree of our satisfaction with a description affects how much we or others feel we know about things. When we are satisfied, things have a reality they do not when we are not satisfied.

This book discusses formal and informal descriptions as they occur in a particular clinical setting, Wilshire Rehabilitation Hospital,* an average-size (92-bed) physical rehabilitation facility. It is primarily concerned with how the hospital's clinical staff select, exchange, and present information concerning physical disability and rehabilitation. Increasingly, clinical staff in this and other settings whose services are paid for by third parties (such as private insurance companies and government agencies) are required to prepare formal written descriptions of the varied features of their ongoing services and responsibilities and how these affect the lives of their clients and patients.

While formal reporting to outside agents has increased in volume and complexity in recent years, service providers have always been, and continue to be, also responsible for describing their services to each other, to their clients, and to the clients' families. Such descriptions are mixtures of casual telling and official reporting. At the hospital under discussion, subject matter ranges from body flexion and return of function to clients' family size and household composition.

Whatever its particular content or mode, the activity of clinical description is taken seriously. Reports range in subject from conditions, such as strokes, spinal cord injury, and amputations, to patient progress in rehabilitation (or "rehab"). While what is described may be more or less formal, more or less concrete, it is nonetheless about things that audiences and describers believe is worth knowing, in which much is at stake, both in terms of health and finances. As a formally organized human service setting, the hospital provides a place for studying the complexities of description, a place where description is about serious matters. It is a setting in which participants are continually concerned with the accuracy and adequacy of description.

This book, then, focuses on two topics: (1) the activity of clinical description as a process; and (2) the aspects of this process in the context of a human service organization, in which people expect services to be provided and come to know of them largely by means of what is said or reported about them. Descriptions are therefore of more than casual concern; specificity is highly valued. The

*The names of places and people have been fictionalized throughout.

clinical realities of the setting—needs, expectations, and procedures of patients and caregivers—are thereby bound up with their
description. The first topic provides a mode of understanding and
interpreting what is observed and executed in the hospital; it offers
a means of making sense of its objects and events. The second topic
permits us to illustrate how descriptively practical is the serious
and "accurate" business of rehabilitation.

THE ACTIVITY OF DESCRIBING

The activity of describing has four important components:
the activities, objects, or events being described; the description
itself; the descriptive circumstance; and the audience that receives
the description. To engage in description is to attend in various
ways to each of the components. Routinely, people make a concerted effort to locate the true objects of their concern. When this
is done successfully, the resulting description is sometimes said to
be "valid." People also attempt to avoid erratic or idiosyncratic
attention to the things being described in order to maintain a
modicum of consistency. Consistent descriptions are sometimes
called "reliable." Those who engage in description—whoever they
are—also take into account various concrete conditions in the
circumstances in which they find themselves describing. Description takes place in a particular context, under particular conditions.
And, whether it is an earlier or a later consideration, people expect
to offer their descriptions to some audience, whom they take into
account in organizing what they know for presentation. Audiences
are relevant to descriptive activity to the extent that they exist in
the minds of those formulating descriptions, whether or not it is
clear who the audiences are or might be.
While the activity of describing revolves around the four components, describers commonly believe that they might, at least
ideally, strive to achieve a quality of description that can be judged
solely on grounds of validity and reliability. For example, it is
evident that research methods textbooks in the social sciences
devote the bulk, if not the whole, of their attention to the first two
components, either ignoring or giving lip-service to the other two.
As they might caution, the quality of description should not be a
matter of circumstance nor audience. Rather, to offer descriptions
and comment on their quality is to attend to the relationship
between the description and that described. The extent to which
this relationship is claimed or judged to be valid and/or reliable is

an indirect warrant for glossing over circumstance and audience. Presumably, an ideal description is only about that described. Indeed, to be a professional clinical describer suggests that one does not permit circumstance and audience to affect quality, which, in turn, is a sign of professionalism.

Much seems to be missing from valid and reliable description. We are left with little or no insight into its practice and cannot judge its quality in that regard. We do not know how its quality is affected by the fact that an audience receives it. We have no way of knowing what images of things described are taken by describers to be the relevant ways of presenting things for particular audiences. These missing components of description are the special focus of this study.

We center our concern on the *practice* of clinical description and the audience-relevant *images* of rehabilitation that serve as the frameworks for the communication and description of the staff's clinical activity. By "practice" we mean the ongoing conceptual, interpersonal, and physical work done by staff as they engage in the activity of communicating and describing (Garfinkel, 1967; Zimmerman and Pollner, 1970; Mehan and Wood, 1975). By "image" is meant the sense of rehabilitation that staff call on to frame their depictions (Schutz, 1962; Berger and Luckmann, 1966; Goffman, 1974). Use of images is intimately tied to audience considerations; how one speaks or writes about things depends on who is spoken or written to. The tie is not conceived purely as dramatic effect. It is equally, if not more basically, a matter of presumed differences in understanding among different audiences with regard to the realities of rehabilitation.

Images

In the practice of assembling and offering descriptions, people are more or less aware that to find out about things in order to inform, they bring their attentions to the task. It seems obvious, perhaps too obvious, that in order to be in receipt of knowledge, one must also bring oneself to bear in the matter. This suggests that, even though we understand that there are things to be known, things separate from us, it is us or others who engage the task. The practical matter of bringing and paying attention to things suggests a course of possibilities, possible images of the way things really are.

In the everyday clinical affairs of Wilshire Hospital and other particular places, people do vary in their orientation to the general issue of the relationship between things and images. At one extreme are those who see images, at best, as trivial impediments to the business of obtaining factual and precise knowledge of things, that is, formulating unbiased descriptions of them. Such persons sometimes are considered to be difficult to work with because they resent having to attend seriously to alternative images that might be brought to bear in the presentation or reception of descriptions. At the other extreme are those who see almost everything in terms of images. They also are sometimes considered to be difficult to work with because they tend "not to be serious about things." Descriptive activity is articulated through the range of persons who have such varying orientations.

Images may be well or poorly delineated. While people make reference to ways of seeing things, the ways are not necessarily recognized as images in their own right. Reference to image is oblique and undeveloped when it is suggested, for example, that a certain report should show evidence that the reporters "have the right things in mind," not bothering to specify the meaning of "right things." On the other hand, some images are well delineated and even named. For example, at Wilshire, it is not uncommon to hear references to the medical image or the "medical model" of rehabilitation. Even though there is variation in the specification of images, in use, all images are vague to some degree. While two or three images of rehabilitation may be well known to certain staff members, it is a continuing practical problem for everyone involved as to which of two or three images (or lesser known ones) should be used in the course of assembling or presenting descriptions.

Audiences and Describers

What is the relationship between audiences, describers, and images? Staff members describe for each other, for outside agents such as insurance companies, for families, and for patients, who, in turn, are the various audiences who may or may not explicitly be taken into account in deciding "how to put things." Clinical team members are centrally engaged in the role of describers because they are considered to be formally and directly responsible for ongoing rehabilitation. However, there are circumstances where families and patients become describers too. For example, patients are the audience under consideration, but family members are the describers when the latter talk over with a patient's social worker how to present a decision about where the patient is to be discharged. Staff members are the audience under consideration when members of different patients' families offer each other advice about, say, how to ask questions of, or get information from, nurses or from certain doctors.

While the problems of description may be anyone's active concern, we focus our attention on how the concern presents itself to staff members as describers in relation to their routine audiences. Among staff members as describers, it may be made fairly explicit which images are believed to be basic in·organizing a written or oral report. Staff members know of and remind each other that, say, for the audience of families, descriptions are framed one way, and for the audience of fellow staff members, they are put another way. Well-known audience variations delimit descriptive activity but they do not determine them. The variations serve describers as *typical* rules-of-thumb, as a routine means of specifying basic images and organizing descriptive actions for ongoing practical purposes.

Describers and audiences have both their formal/informal and their practical organization. Formally, certain team members are responsible for doing evaluations of a patient's physical disability soon after admission, and relevant staff members are expected to participate in the team conferences. They periodically participate in family conferences where they present reports about the patient to family members. The obligations designate formal audiences. In addition, there are informal connections between describers and audiences. For example, it is known that certain doctors are helpful in deciding "what to say" to families while other doctors are not, some of them relying on the therapists for their own descriptive needs. In practice the knowledge of variation in formal and informal describer-audience relationships is a resource used in the service of specifying whether, or what, particular images might be taken into account in description.

The relationship between images and audiences is both definite and tenuous. It is definite in that there are working beliefs about how particular audiences approach things, about the particular images they· have of things. For example, it is "known" that families are likely to see things in ways that staff members do not. The knowledge informs staff members of how to approach family members with information about patient progress and the like. But staff members also tacitly accept the knowledge as *working* information, tentative knowledge about a concrete descriptive condition. For example, a belief that informs staff members that families have a particular image of physical rehabilitation suggests to staff members that they assemble a particular kind of description of it for a family conference. But when someone mentions that, say, the most responsible family member is a nurse, a role quite familiar to staff members, is this particular family to be treated as a typical family audience or is it not? Treating this and other families as "typical" confirms the audience rule for image selection. But so do exceptions. Treating this particular family as an exception implies the existence of a general rule by which to specify the image basic to the descriptive activity.

In practice, audiences, describers, and images have a working relationship—one that integrates and articulates both typical rules and tenuous exception. While it is believed that particular images are best used with select audiences, in any ongoing descriptive activity varying conditions subject the belief to question. The issue is not always resolvable. At times describers admit that they "just don't know how [someone] will react." They may simply conclude that they'll have to take their chances. However, staff members' routine work with each other, with families, with patients, and indirectly with outside agents, informs them that it is, for all practical purposes, safe to assume that an audience is addressed within the purview of a particular image of disability and rehabilitation. In their ongoing validation, image/audience rules produce and reproduce particular descriptions for specific audiences.

Descriptive "Goodness"

Underpinning the practical question of what to say or write to whom is the issue of what constitutes a "good" description. In principle a good description is one that precisely and consistently reflects what it claims. Being in receipt of such a description is to have knowledge of activities and events as they are. But at the same time, because it is always someone or other who assembles description and someone or other who receives it, it is these people who pass judgment on descriptive "goodness."

Issue may be taken with the "goodness" of a description in its own right, separate from audience considerations. For example, one staff member may remind another in a conference that what seemed to be passing as a finished report is really incomplete or unclear in a number of ways. Or, at a clinical team conference, when a therapist reads from a Progress Note that a patient has made considerable advances since the last conference, and another therapist reads from a note that little or no progress is being made in a closely related area and recommends discharge, discussion is generated over the apparent contradiction.

The "goodness" of descriptions in their own right is distinguished from what may or may not be "good enough" for particular audiences. In the first example, while the finished report seems complete to most of those attending the conference, one participant reminds the rest that the report is really incomplete. In the second example, staff members recognize that a description which they are compiling for a complete written report is not going to be consistent if left as is. The examples provide two important criteria by which descriptive goodness is judged: completeness and consistency (reliability).

Describers work to resolve issues of descriptive "goodness." They attempt to have something to say, should the need arise, in order to sound like they know what they are talking about. They make use of a variety of personal and commonly available techniques to complete descriptions. They take the time, sometimes considerable time, to make sure their descriptions are not contradictory. The work involved in each of these activities is part of the practice of assembling good description.

Descriptive Adequacy

The quality of description also is evaluated in terms of how it relates in image and credibility to particular audiences. Describers may be concerned with whether a description will sound credible to an audience even though its substance is considered to be in line with the audience's ostensible image of things. Audiences may prefer to hear select reports about things because certain ones sound more credible. Image and credibility are features of the adequacy of description. Descriptive adequacy is an audience-oriented quality, in which the working question is: Descriptive goodness *for whom*? Being "good" and adequate suggests that a description is not only consistent and complete but that it is believed to be credibly coherent with an audience's image.

Adequacy is affected by presumed perceptions of describer competence. It is commonly assumed at Wilshire that certain audiences, especially families and third parties, value expert/professional description over nonprofessional description, though this is certainly not unique to the hospital. The assumption is of course subject to practical interpretation. For example, in some specific circumstance, a typical expert, such as a physiatrist, may be considered to be less expert than a particular physical therapist because the physiatrist is reported to have "hardly even seen the patient," while the therapist knows the patient well. But as a working principle, expertise still serves as a credibility rule in the matter of adequacy, as it does in many organizations.

The credibility of any kind of description is affected by how well the description is "backed up." Wilshire staff members believe that while they may know how to speak to families, they are likely to be most convincing when they separate out and refer to some of what they report to families as "data." Whatever is called "data" is objective to the extent that what is convincingly presented reflects disability and rehabilitation, not the describers who speak or write of them.

Not all data seem to be of equal quality in matters of credibility. While Wilshire people believe, in principle, that expert description is desirable and that description supported by data is more convincing than opinion, quantitative (hard) data seem more precise, concise, and concrete than qualitative (soft) data (Gubrium and Buckholdt, 1979). Even though hard data may have to be translated into plain English for an audience, an apparent translation is more credible than plain description. Together with image considerations, credibility sets the practical standard for descriptive adequacy.

THE PARTICIPANTS

A wide range of people participate in the ongoing affairs of care and treatment at Wilshire Hospital. They include patients and their families; the clinical staff—which includes physicians; physical, occupational, speech, and leisure therapists; and social workers—and supporting personnel, such as admitting clerks and medical record secretaries. Others are less directly involved but still enter into everyday hospital affairs in ways that are recognizable to patients and staff members. They include referring physicians and social workers in other institutions, such as acute care hospitals and nursing homes; third-party payers of hospital care, such as private insurance companies and Medicare; and relevant others in and about points of patient entry and discharge, such as relatives and managers of boarding homes.

Most patients at Wilshire suffer incapacities arising from cerebral vascular accidents (CVAs) or stroke, in which the most incapacitating symptoms are aphasia and paralysis. Another prevalent condition is spinal cord injury (SCI); its incapacities vary from quadriplegia (near to full, permanent paralysis of the four extremities) to paraparesis (partial paralysis of the lower extremities). A third condition is head trauma, commonly the result of diving or automobile accidents, with its various complications. Other conditions include amputation, hip fracture, multiple sclerosis, arthritis, hip replacement, and a host of less commonly encountered physical problems, such as those associated with ankylosing spondylosis and brain stem infarction. The purpose of the hospital is to treat patients whose physical incapacities are associated with these conditions.

Among the staff are a number of persons who process the patient through the hospital. Admissions officers receive and distribute incoming documents to various staff members who evaluate them. One of the main tasks is determination of whether referrals are appropriate candidates for physical rehab. Those involved in the evaluation include: a nurse who serves as an admissions reviewer, the heads of physical and occupational therapy departments, and individual physicians on the admissions committee. When a patient is admitted, he or she is assigned to a social worker, who is responsible for mediating family-staff relations and planning the patient's eventual discharge from the hospital. (The average length of stay is four to six weeks.) The nurse who serves as admissions reviewer also coordinates the hospital's utilization review, in which the patient's hospital stay is monitored for whether it continues to be justifiable. Medical record and unit secretaries manage the flow of documented information. And, finally, escort aides deliver patients to and from therapeutic services.

Officially the central therapeutic department at Wilshire is physical therapy (PT). A patient's problem must require physical therapy to justify admission and stay. Beyond PT, a patient's condition may indicate a need for occupational therapy (OT), speech therapy, and psychological services. Each ,of these four services requires a physician's order, and each is billed separately. As part of their hospital stay, patients receive nursing care and are assigned an attending physician from the hospital's medical staff, which includes physiatrists, neurologists, internists, and family physicians. The services of three leisure therapists and two pastoral counselors are also available to patients. The hospital makes use of consulting psychiatrists, cardiologists, and specialists in relevant areas of physical medicine as needed.

In briefly describing the kinds of physical conditions that come within the purview of care at Wilshire and the range of services offered and available, we have borrowed heavily from official designations. Officially, Wilshire is a hospital; officially, it specializes in the rehabilitation of physical disabilities; officially, it provides a number of therapeutic services. Official description is thus used by staff members when they are asked, directly or indirectly, to describe for what and how a speciality hospital such as this one provides care. It is found in the documents that summarize the hospital's services for interested publics, such as the brochures sent to families who wish to know whether Wilshire can help their relatives and to the institutions that might refer patients to Wilshire. It is the material of reports of hospital activities and applications filed with regulating agencies, such as hospital accreditation boards and professional standards review organizations.

Wilshire's clinical activities are described in still other ways. Referring physicians in acute care hospitals sometimes designate the patients' problems as largely custodial—medically untreatable—and Wilshire's therapeutic services as mainly evaluatory, an intermediate stage in the general interinstitutional processing of the physically handicapped. What takes place at the rehabilitation hospital is thus portrayed as "not really" hospital activity but something perhaps midway between curing and custody. Indeed, on occasion, an outside physician's referral will cast Wilshire as a convalescent center or nursing home. In contrast to this, other descriptions by referring physicians, families, and patients portray Wilshire as a superhospital where the patient is referred for treatment after he is discharged from an acute care hospital because "nothing more can be done" for him. A family may have sought admission to Wilshire for an elderly father because they expect him to be, as they might put it, "normal again in time and like he used to be." They see Wilshire as that hospital where one continues what was begun in an acute care setting where the father was taken immediately after his stroke.

Rehabilitation. Evaluation. Custody. Cure. These are four different terms by which to describe the clinical activities of Wilshire personnel. As we shall show in Chapter 2, entire frameworks or sets of images exist for each of the terms. While staff are held responsible for using the official mode to describe their work, they also recognize and speak the language of the other descriptions and images of hospital therapeutic activity. Staff members are able to describe patient problems and the hospital's therapeutic efforts in ways that are not completely compatible with each other, some of which would be officially unrecognizable.

CLINICAL ROUTINE

Description of clinical activity by staff emerges from daily routine and its ongoing practical contingencies. At the same time, the routine is the working stuff of description. The following is a more or less formal chronology of the routine.

Patients are ordinarily awakened between 6:45 and 7:15 A.M. on weekdays by their primary nurses, who provide most of the routine personal and nursing care at Wilshire, although aides sometimes assist. Each nurse is assigned two to four patients, depending on the level of care. The nursing supervisor on a unit helps if a nurse is ill or on vacation. Since certain therapies are scheduled in the patient's room from 8 to 9 A.M., there is some rush to have these patients ready. Some patients are alert and mobile enough to eat breakfast on their own; they may dine in their rooms or move to the outer courts on which all rooms exit. Other patients must be fed by the nurse. They may also have to be cleaned up and dressed. Between 8:00 and 8:30 A.M., most patients have eaten and are dressed for their daily activities. If they are not bedridden, they are asked to vacate their rooms so the nurse can change the bedding and tidy up. Some move on their own; others are pushed in their wheelchairs to the outside court or to 9:00 A.M. therapy appointments, if such have been scheduled.

Many of the fifteen occupational therapists begin seeing patients in the latter's rooms between 8:00 and 8:30 A.M. These early appointments are referred to as "floor ADLs" or "bed ADLs" (activities of daily living). An OT may have additional ADL sessions later in the day. In bed ADLs, the therapist teaches the patient how to be mobile in bed, to sit up, to swing one's legs over the side, and to get in and out of bed safely and efficiently; these activities may also include getting into and out of a wheelchair and using the bathroom. Floor ADLs generally refers to the teaching of dressing skills. In ADL sessions occurring later in the day, patients are taught personal hygiene and eating techniques ("feeding ADLs"), the latter during lunch. The later ADLs may or may not be conducted in the patient's room.

While only some patients have ADL appointments, almost all participate at some time during the day in functional OT. At 9:00 A.M. each of the occupational therapists begins to work with individual patients for thirty-minute periods in a large room called the OT clinic. The functional program, which includes a variety of range-of-motion exercises for the hands, arms, and shoulders, is designed to increase the strength and function of the upper body.

To "range" a limb is to exercise it over the full range of flexible motion. Functional OT is scheduled from 9:00 to 11:30 A.M. and, after a lunch break, continues from 1:00 to 3:00 P.M. or thereabouts. In addition to ADLs and functional activities, the OT department works with some patients on homemaking and work simplification skills, makes splints and other adaptive devices, and conducts classes in avocational activities (handicrafts, for example), cooking, adaptive living (bedmaking, for example), and functional hand skills (such as typing).

Physical therapy has a schedule much like OT except that while all Wilshire therapists report to work at 8:00 A.M., PTs generally do not begin seeing patients until 9:00 A.M. The fifteen PTs offer several services, the most prominent of which are exercise and gait training. Both focus on the hips and/or legs since, in the hospital division of labor, the PT's area of expertise centers on the rehabilitation of the lower extremities. Exercise involves working individually with a patient for 30-minute periods each day on some aspect of lower body functioning. Gait training takes several forms. If a patient needs to relearn how to walk, a therapist will do the teaching and supervise practice for an additional thirty minutes each day. If the problem is lower extremity weakness and the need for support and monitoring because of bad safety techniques in walking, a PT aide is assigned to supervise gait training. For those patients more advanced in skill and strength and needing only additional practice, an aide, but sometimes a therapist, supervises a gait class for up to an hour each day, usually in the afternoon. PT also offers pelvic and cervical traction, postural drainage, and a variety of "special modalities," such as hot and cold packs, ultraviolet treatments, diathermy, hydrotherapy, paraffin baths, biofeedback, transcutaneous nerve stimulation, and ultrasound. Along with OT, PT makes home visits in order to assess the kinds of mobility and safety problems the patient might encounter when he returns home, such as steep stairways or doorways too narrow for a wheelchair to pass.

Unlike PT and OT, which provide services to virtually all patients on a daily basis, speech therapy is administered to only about a fourth of the patients, who participate in 30-minute sessions ranging from twice daily to every other day. Although speech difficulties as such are not justifiable grounds for admission, speech therapy may be recommended by a therapist and ordered by a physician once a person is admitted for physical rehabilitation. Unlike her counterparts in PT and OT, the head of the speech department has a regular patient load, as do the other two speech therapists. Patients may need help in two major areas. One involves the physical apparatus of speech, including oral musculature, breath control, movement of the tongue, and the like. The other focuses on the cognitive processing needed for communication—the abilities to comprehend incoming stimuli and to respond in appropriate and meaningful ways (receptive and expressive skills, respectively). Most of the speech therapists' time is spent in evaluating and working to improve cognitive functioning.

At some point during the day, usually in the morning, the patient is visited by a doctor. Seven staff physicians and residents in physiatry are responsible for daily medical care and supervision. One of them, an internist, is designated chief of staff. He handles the largest patient load, between twenty and twenty-five, and has the additional responsibility of overseeing a variety of management or administrative tasks. The other six doctors list their specialities as general surgery and medicine, neurology, general practice, internal medicine, medicine and surgery, and physiatry. The medical staff includes two other physiatrists. One is the chief of the Department of Physical Medicine and Rehabilitation at the hospital and head of the same department at a nearby medical school; his services are limited to general matters of policy and procedure, occasionally making determinations in disagreements among staff on matters of admission and discharge, and infrequent consultation. The other physiatrist primarily conducts neurophysiological studies, although he sometimes substitutes for physicians who are ill or on vacation. He also conducts weekly orthotic clinics, where patients are evaluated for appliances such as leg braces.

Patients also have contact with social workers, although less regularly and frequently than with nurses, therapists, or physicians. The Social Service Department employs five social workers, one of whom is designated as the head. They meet with each patient or his family soon after admission and begin planning for the patient's life after discharge, including living arrangements, care and supervision, outpatient services, and the return to work or the development of other interests. Social workers also arrange conferences for patient, family, and clinical staff during the patient's stay, at which staff members report on the patient's progress and family members discuss their own aims, needs, and expected problems. Involvement in more day-to-day aspects of patients' lives may also occur. For example, if a patient seems overly depressed or hostile, a social worker may attempt some counseling. Social workers assist patients in a variety of ways. A social worker may help a patient contact a lawyer or inquire about a disability check that has not arrived. At Wilshire the social work staff also participate in three support groups: one for patients who have suffered spinal cord injury, one for their families, and one for the families of stroke patients.

Morning and afternoon life at Wilshire is busy for most patients. Although a few may be confined temporarily to their rooms because of medical complications, most are up and about from early morning until late afternoon. With regular appointments with the various therapists, movement from one therapy session to another, and meals, they are usually involved in some scheduled activity. Even nonscheduled periods may be filled with visits from the doctor, a social worker, or family members. What little free time there is during the day is spent watching television on two central courts, chatting with other patients, resting in one's room, or participating in some activity sponsored by leisure services.

Therapists are also busy. Most of them have appointments with patients every thirty minutes over the entire working day, except during lunch. They have "breaks" only if a patient cannot or will not come to therapy or if the hospital census declines. Whatever free time they do have may be spent writing patient progress notes or completing patient evaluation forms, activities that sometimes spill over into lunch break. In addition, they may be scheduled to attend a team or family conference or go on a home visit. When substitutes cannot be found, frequent scheduling conflicts result in the cancellation of patient appointments.

By 4:00 P.M., the hospital is a much less active place; except for nurses, most of the clinical staff have left. While a few may return in the evening to participate in support groups, and leisure services is busy with evening activities, after 4 P.M. Wilshire has the "ward-look" of any ordinary hospital or nursing home. The smaller nursing staff attend to evening needs and other patient care business, such as occasionally taking blood pressure, measuring urine output, and monitoring bowel movements. During evening hours little therapeutic work is expected of patients; they relax and rest for the next day's round of activities or visit with family or friends. What distinguishes Wilshire as an institution specializing in physical rehabilitation takes place mainly on weekdays, from 8 A.M. to 4 P.M..

Chapter 2

Images and the Descriptive Process

The manner in which Wilshire people communicate with each other and outsiders about rehabilitation includes both general and specific references to clinical routine. But the descriptive activity also includes attention to the object of or audiences for this activity, within the framework of select images. Images, or possible depictions of the way things are, provide frameworks for describing rehabilitation.

At Wilshire, communication and description by clinical staff range in subject from the progress of a particular patient to the place of a rehabilitation hospital in the health care delivery system. In this chapter we consider some prominent images that enter into descriptions of rehabilitation. Here, for analytic purposes, we separate images and audiences and focus on images, in order to show the range and types available for descriptive work. In the next chapters, we will demonstrate how staff members bring these resources to bear as they engage in practical description in specific situations.

IMAGES OF PLACE

Wilshire presents and elicits different images to different people, and sometimes to the same person. What sort of place does

Wilshire seem to be? Officially it is a hospital, but it is both more and less than that. It is also an educational center; much of its work is spoken of as teaching and learning. In some respects it is a nursing home; some patients are said to need only custodial care. It is occasionally described in terms of what it originally was (from before the turn of the century until the early sixties)—a sanitarium —a kind of semi-spa where the well-heeled took their rest and sought "the treatment." What Wilshire, the place, actually *is* therefore varies from one circumstance or audience to another and is articulated by means of images.

The Hospital Image

Many events identify Wilshire as a hospital. Nurses perform the daily bed-and-body work common to all hospitals. They dispense medication, give injections, clean bladder or bowel "accidents," and feed or bathe patients. Many at Wilshire believe that their nursing care is better than in most hospitals in that patients generally have the attention of a single primary care nurse for all their cares on a shift. Doctors make daily rounds. The doctors spend a few minutes with each patient, chatting, listening to complaints, examining, and ordering medications and tests. Other obvious signs that this is a hospital include nursing stations, patient charts, oxygen tanks, intravenous paraphernalia, and a public address system on which doctors and other members of the clinical staff are paged.

While Wilshire is certainly a hospital in some respects, it does not offer all the services available in an acute care facility. For example, it does not have emergency or surgical services. Ambulances do not rush here, carrying victims of car crashes, heart attacks, or physical assault. If anything, ambulances quietly leave Wilshire to deliver medically unstable patients *to* acute care hospitals; if time is insufficient, a paramedic unit is called to deliver emergency treatment at the scene. Patients are also sent to other hospitals for particular tests that are more or less routine in an ordinary hospital. Thus Wilshire is less than a hospital in some ways.

In other respects, however, it is seen as a hospital of last resort. While patients with acute problems may be discharged to other hospitals until their medical problems are "stabilized" and then can resume their therapeutic programs at Wilshire, this is not always the case. At times doctors may feel that the primary nursing at Wilshire provides much better care and supervision than at an ordinary hospital and that a patient should remain here, unless an unusual emergency arises, even though he or she cannot participate in therapy.

The availability of an extensive range of therapies is another way Wilshire stands above most other hospitals, at least for the particular kinds of patients it treats. While many hospitals have speech, physical and occupational therapy, and related services, it is generally felt by the staff that the emphasis on and quality of these services at Wilshire renders them superior to their counterparts in acute care facilities that play a comparatively minor role.

The School Image

With no surgical or other conventional medical departments, such as obstetrics, psychiatry, and orthopedics, what constitutes "medical" treatment at Wilshire? While in many ways the place looks like a hospital and is seen or presented that way, treatment is not primarily medical or surgical.

Another image of Wilshire is as an educational institution, in which the most important activities are communicated and described in terms of teaching and learning. Doctors, for example, sometimes invoke this image when they discharge patients to an acute care hospital. If their medical conditions preclude participation in physical rehabilitation, patients are told that they can return when they are well enough to learn. The hospital administrator also recognizes the legitimacy of the educational image. He once mounted an unsuccessful campaign to describe this function in choosing the name of the institution, something like "Wilshire Rehabilitation and Educational Institute"; (many rehabilitation hospitals are officially called "institutes.") The board of directors vetoed the move, apparently anticipating trouble with third-party payers and community contributors who see Wilshire as a hospital. Wilshire is in fact accredited as a hospital.

The educational image is probably most prominent for the hospital therapists. As they often state, teaching and learning, not medical work, constitute the hospital's central functions. On occasion, in conversations, they express amusement or resentment over the fact that while doctors are normally in charge of the hospital, they know very little about rehabilitation. This attitude extends to one of the two nonadministrative physiatrists on the staff who is said to be more interested in his so-called studies than treatment. As one physical therapist commented:

They tell us to do something for the patients, somehow make them better. They don't tell us what to do or how to do it. We do all the work and they just sign the papers saying it's been done. Except for the minor medical problems, I don't think we need them.

Whether this view takes the form of amusement or resentment depends on the circumstance. It is sometimes amusing, for example, when doctors admit their ignorance or indirectly rely on the therapists for particular judgments. Resentment emerges, sometimes openly, when medical interests interfere with teaching and learning. For example, therapists are frustrated and become angry when patients are admitted who cannot benefit from therapy and they must "waste their time" trying to work with them. They become particularly vexed when patients are admitted because they are considered medically "interesting" by a staff physician, though not in terms of any functional disability.

The contrast between the medical and the educational image stands out clearly when staff members openly discuss how they generally deal with those in their care. In some instances they are called "patients"; in others, "clients" seems like a better choice. The distinction is not maintained along purely professional lines, with doctors always seeing "patients" and therapists working with "clients." On occasion, doctors remind therapists they have *clients* whose needs go beyond the medical arena. In turn, therapists present physicians with *patient* problems, which are medical rather than purely educational. The image changes as situations arise which seem to call for one image or the other.

Explicit references to patients or clients as such are not as important, however, as the more general understanding of the relevance of the medical or educational image in a particular circumstance. For example, when clinical staff members met to discuss the status of a middle-aged stroke victim who had developed an infection, a therapist complained that the patient was not yet strong enough to benefit from therapy. The doctor agreed and suggested that while daily work with the patient should continue, they should not expect much therapeutic progress. He told them that when the medical problem was sufficiently stabilized, they "could begin thinking of him as a client rather than a patient." On another occasion, several therapists were pressuring a doctor to release a particular patient. They argued that this person had received all possible benefits from therapy and that no further improvements could be expected. While doctors usually accept such recommendations from therapists, in this case the physician balked, informing the therapists that the patient still had medical problems that "needed looking into" and lecturing them about their failure to see the hospital as anything more than a rehabilitation setting.

Continual tension exists between the hospital and school images of Wilshire as a place of treatment. While both medical and educational images are pervasive and are more or less recognized by staff members, it is not always clear which image is at stake or will serve as an adequate framework for describing activities. This tension is only resolved in practice.

Well-known rules-of-thumb indicate the ways in which particular audiences hold particular images of the facility. For example, the "public" is sometimes said typically to hold a hospital image of Wilshire which, according to some therapists, occasionally makes it difficult to describe what is, or what can be, accomplished in treatment. But such typical descriptions of what occurs at Wilshire are subject to the interpretive contingencies of everyday practice. Who constitutes "the public"? If it is understood as an audience of families with members who have been referred to Wilshire for further medical treatment, the medical image is focal. If, on the other hand, the public is a television audience concerned with how stroke victims and the spinal-cord injured can be taught to adapt to their disabilities, the educational image is in the forefront. (Such a program was actually filmed at Wilshire.) The descriptive tension over the varied concerns and activities of Wilshire Hospital's clinical regimen revolves around practical questions of clinical reality, typical images of different audiences who receive the descriptions, and who the audience is considered to be in a particular situation.

The Nursing Home Image

Another image of Wilshire is that of a nursing home. While staff members dislike the image, they sometimes use it in regard to some patients without acute medical problems who lack rehabilitation goals or possibilities. They often are older persons and persons who staff feel should be discharged but have no satisfactory residential alternative. They cannot survive on their own, and for a variety of reasons, they cannot be discharged to a family home or to a nursing facility. Therapeutic goals are often invented for such persons to justify a longer stay at Wilshire, but staff is in general agreement that they cannot remain for long if only custodial care is needed. While such individuals are often discharged within one or two weeks after the staff decide that nothing more can be done for them at Wilshire, at least a few persons remain in the informal status of receiving temporary custodial care. Thus the nursing home image becomes a viable alternative to the medical and educational images of place in descriptive practice.

The nursing home image emerges not only—or primarily—from the staff understanding of exigency and need inside Wilshire. Some families and outside professionals think of Wilshire as custodial or, as one social worker put it, "like a real good nursing home —something that no one around here really likes to hear." Just before the start of an evening support group for families of stroke victims, a participant described Wilshire to a first-timer as "...sort of like a nursing home with a big P.T. department. They [patients] get out, though, and they do do good work here." Staff take great pains, both in oral presentation to families and written reports to agents, such as outside professionals and third-party payers, to highlight the therapeutic features of Wilshire services—lest Wilshire be thought to be nothing more than a fine nursing home, which, among other consequences, might result in bad publicity, raise questions of superfluous staff, and lead to retroactive nonpayment of services.

The Sanitarium Image

A fourth image of Wilshire is as a sanitarium. It had been called a sanitarium for about one hundred years prior to the sixties, when it became a rehabilitation hospital. Wealthy persons and celebrities from around the country once came here to rest and regain their physical and psychological health. Except for an elegantly appointed recreation and meeting room, most signs of plush residential living are now gone. A new one-story structure houses all patients and is the center for all therapy except speech which, at the time of this study, was located in one of two older structures. (Speech was soon moved to the new building.) The administrative offices, medical records, pharmacy, cafeteria, doctors' offices, and several other nonclinical departments are located in the older structures but, judging from old photographs, the luxuriousness of the old institution has been stripped away or underplayed. Patients are rarely seen in the older buildings unless on their way to or from speech therapy or the cafeteria. With the movement of most clinical activities to the new building and the modifications of the older structures, the physical appearance of the hospital is now dominated more by brick, glass, concrete, and acoustical tile than by mahogany woodwork, hardwood floors, arched entries, mosaic tiling, and tapestries. The difference is not merely architectural, however; it has been accompanied by clientele changes, the medicalization of problems and services, and the professionalization of the clinical staff.

The change in physical appearance has not totally eliminated the image of the hospital as a sanitarium, however. The director of public relations mentions his perennial difficulty in communicating the relatively new image of a rehabilitation hospital to the public and to the medical profession: "When people hear Wilshire, they still say, 'Oh yes, the sanitarium.'" It is said that some persons who are eligible and in need of rehabilitation services either never think of Wilshire or reject it because of the former image. Who can afford "the cure" or "water treatment"—activities now referred to as "rehabilitation" and "hydrotherapy," respectively? The old image also causes some fund-raising difficulty. A sanitarium for the rich is not exactly a public institution and people are not yet fully aware of the wide range of services available to the public in a rehabilitation hospital—services covered by various public and private insurance plans.

The old image of the sanitarium also lingers within the daily routine of the hospital. Therapists recommend and doctors prescribe hot packs, compresses, or whirlpool baths for, as they say, "psychological reasons." While these treatments may or may not be seen as contributing directly to progress, they help the patient relax sufficiently to be in the mood to benefit from the therapist's efforts. These treatments are also sometimes suggested for patients who complain that nothing is being done for them or that they are not improving. Some therapists compare these treatments with a trip to a mineral spring or attendance at a revival meeting. If a patient has faith in their healing powers, who can say that they might not work? While therapists themselves have little confidence in the restorative powers of treatments that are not focused on the hard work required for genuine rehabilitation, they are generally quite willing to allow patients to believe in and have access to them as long as they participate in regular rehabilitative programs.

Staff members believe that for patients who are resting or convalescing, the institution is functioning much more like a sanitarium or nursing home, respectively, than a hospital. While they often do not approve of this and complain of inappropriate admissions, they feel that improvement or lack of improvement in some cases has little to do with their therapeutic efforts. As a sanitarium, the hospital is a convenient and pleasant place to be as time passes and events unfold, as one doctor and several therapists speak of it—a hotel with its guests, a place where persons stay and are in certain respects taken care of until they feel ready to return home or move on to some other more suitable place of residence.

IMAGES OF TREATMENT

Surrounding and interwoven with daily clinical routine are images that deal not so much with the nature of Wilshire as a place as with the work that is undertaken in the name of physical rehabilitation. Ideally staff and others believe that the hospital's aim is to return patients to a state of normal living. However, there are various ways of seeing what is done on behalf of the goal as well as differing perspectives on what the goal means in particular instances. These are images of treatment and its effects—means of interpreting and presenting the nature of the rehabilitation process.

Professional Treatment

Early photographs of Wilshire and its staff when it was a sanitarium reveal several contrasts with the present. In addition to the physical differences already noted, there is a difference in the appearance of staff. Formerly, nuns were in charge of the institution; they staffed the administration, provided the nursing care, and offered patients therapeutic rest, relaxation, and exercise. Today nuns are not visible in the daily routine of the hospital, except in the dining hall where a few, mainly nonclinical sisters, eat together. They rarely interact with patients or staff.

Staff members occasionally express amusement over the former character of the institution and what it represented. It was not as professional a setting as it now is, with staff specifically trained and certified for their functions. The contrast surfaces whenever the history and quality of the institution is discussed. For example, the hospital recently held a fund-raising dinner where a former administrative nun was invited to be keynote speaker. She talked of the importance of Christian love, understanding, and kindness in rehabilitation work. The following day, several PTs and OTs took issue with part of her message. While they did not reject its Christian love aspect, they scoffed at its lack of attention to expertise, and speculated that the speaker's inability to "keep up with the times" probably led to her and her order's demise at the hospital. Similar sentiments circulate about the hospital's former chief administrator, who was also a nun. Current staff members who remember her resented her unwillingness to accord professional training in physical rehabilitation the status it deserved, and they speak of her overbearing interference in what were properly matters of professional judgment.

The importance of professional skill and autonomy was the topic of considerable bickering and resentment by several therapists when the hospital was visited by a motion picture celebrity. As part of its ongoing effort to inform the public, potential donors, and public officials of the hospital's services and the therapeutic value of physical medicine and rehabilitation, the hospital arranged for a local television interview show to be produced at the hospital, with a now-recovered celebrity reporting on her well-known experiences with stroke and her dramatic comeback. After the interview several therapists spoke disparagingly about the way the celebrity described her recovery. She gave glowing credit to understanding, private-duty nurses and an attentive husband who "stuck close by her" and arranged a continuing parade of friends and relatives to visit her *at home*. Indeed, at one point in the interview, when she was asked about how she reacted to her helplessness, she said that she "just couldn't be hospitalized because it was just too, too embarrassing," but that, with the help of her friends, she managed a near-perfect recovery. She then emphasized to her television audience that they too should have hope, for they also could recover from stroke to once again lead normal and full lives. The Wilshire therapists who heard this concluded that either she did not remember the value of the professional help she had received or her strokes had been relatively mild ones. If they had been severe, it is doubtful she could ever have recovered without professional attention.

Physical, occupational, and speech therapists each claim particular expertise in physical rehabilitation. They speak technical languages that refer to muscle function, nerve pathways, anatomy, skeletal structure, and parts of the brain. They evaluate patients upon admission and just before discharge. During the patient's stay, each formulates and provides more or less standard therapeutic programs. They speak of stages of physical recovery and the expected psychological features of the several stages. While physicians have formal authority over many decisions regarding patients, they defer to the therapists in all but strictly medical matters. Informally, therapists believe that they know much more about rehabilitation than the doctors do, with the possible excep-

tion of an attending physiatrist, and that they do the most significant clinical work at the hospital. They resent patients and families who give credit for recovery to a doctor. It is, after all, the
application of their expert skills, guided by their professional judgment, that is central to physical rehabilitation.

The social workers, too, consider themselves an important component of the professional team. While they do not participate
directly in physical rehabilitation and have little specialized training in the area, their advice is sought on numerous occasions and
they have input regarding numerous professional decisions. For
example, if therapists feel that a patient has received maximum
benefit from treatments offered and recommend immediate discharge, the actual discharge may be delayed until the patient's
social worker locates and arranges a discharge destination. Most
staff members agree that a professional rehabilitation program
requires attention to the psychosocial and familial dimensions of
recovery, and social workers now consider themselves full-fledged
members of the professional rehabilitation team. They once complained that their full professional status as team partners was not
borne out in the patient's chart; summaries of social service interviews with the patient and his family were not included along with
other service reports. In recognition of their professional function,
their summaries were eventually regularly placed in the charts,
and they contain information on rehabilitation goals as seen by
the patient and the family, a patient's former roles in the family
and community, the impact of the disability on the patient and
the family, education-vocational-avocational attainments and interests, financial resources, discharge plans, and social service
goals.

The professional image of treatment pervades all clinical departments, is manifested in various ways, and is evident in the names
assigned to the various services provided, names that emulate the
public recognition of the medical profession. OTs and PTs are
called "therapists" and their clinical activity is embodied in "treatments." Speech therapists are officially recognized as "speech
pathologists." Members of the department of leisure services refer
to themselves as "leisure therapists", "recreation therapists", or
"activity therapists", the precise name they assign themselves not
yet crystallized. The staff psychologists are "clinical psychologists" and are sent a select number of patients for psychothera-
peutic consults (assessments, testing, counseling). Social workers,
too, see themselves as professional clinicians and would like to
devote more of their time to individual counseling but complain

of the continual press of people-processing duties that prevent them from realizing this important component of their expertise. With the exception of leisure services, the departments also manifest a professional image in standardized professional reports and regular participation in professional team conferences with doctors and nurses (the latter being traditional members of the medical team).

The clearest case of the value of the professional image of treatment at Wilshire is evidenced in the desire for professional recognition by the leisure services staff. The director of the department continually campaigns for presence by members of her department in the various clinical affairs of the hospital. Aside from a very limited number of leisure consultations, suggested but not ordered by doctors, leisure service activities are largely composed of what the department prefers to call "therapeutic recreation": wheelchair games, group exercise classes on weekends, evening card games and crossword puzzle sessions, dinner and entertainment outings. The director resents being forced to merely "fill in" the patient care gaps left by OT, PT, speech, and nursing. As she explained:

> Sometimes they call this the "activities department"...like in nursing homes. But we're really more than that. The leisure services we provide are more than just a time-filler. I mean we're not just here to fill in the patient's time when OT and PT are done with him. There's a real sense in which we provide an important service to the patient, for when he or she is going to leave this place. They're going to have a heck of a lot of leisure time on their hands and they're going to have to *learn* to *fill* it or use it. Leisure, to these people, is going to mean more than just what you do after work or when your work is over. I mean, you know, that's what their work is going to be in a very real sense—leisure is what they're going to have to do. So we get involved in teaching them how to fill their leisure time. It's a therapeutic orientation. We've all been trained in leisure, or actually, recreation therapy. A lot of activity people in nursing homes have had no formal training at all. They just fill in those departments with whoever they can get.
>
> Now that's kind of an ideal picture I'm giving you of what we do here. Patients who have had strokes or spinal injuries often think this leisure stuff is just a lark...something to fill in time here until they get better to leave and resume a former way of life. It just doesn't sink into many of them that their lives are going to be different when they get out, that they're going to have a hell of a lot of time on their hands. Not all react that way of course, but many do. And, you know, they don't start thinking about that until two or three weeks before discharge when, all of a sudden, the light bulb goes on...they learn

that the leisure thing is something they better be more serious about. But, as you can see, right after admission, we don't seem to get much of anywhere with many of them.

The director of leisure services spoke at length about "what leisure services could be," about her image of "a really professional service." It is evident that an ideal leisure service department should be, above all, a professional service with its own language and expertise and be recognized as such, much like PT and OT.

In this place [Wilshire], I can tell you right away what the status ladder is. PTs are the big deals in the place. OT wants to be just like PT and tries to organize all their therapists around power-building exercises and stuff like that. And RT [recreation therapy (leisure services)] is sort of OT's little cousin. We're assigned to do all the "activities"...I hate that word...all the activities that OT wants to get away from, the stuff that used to be called "diversional therapy." So they think that leisure services is just for passing time, you know, filling in the gaps, so to speak. The other thing is that we're thought of as the "avoc"—avocational—department. OT likes to label recreation "avoc," which means without vocation.

I wrestle with all this all the time. All the RTs do. I mean I really don't know what our function is at Wilshire. I'd like to see leisure services move in a more therapeutic direction because that's the way I see it. We know that patients have real recreational needs and we really think that something can be done for them. OT just doesn't have the skills to work with people recreationally. They just fall all over each other when they're trying to put on a program....

I really think that OT is doing too much that rightfully should be in our territory. We should be doing a lot of the things OTs are doing and billing for. The way we're set up now, we don't get any consults because we're not recognized by anyone as therapeutic. Our aim now across the country is to get the AMA to recognize us as therapeutic. Of course, the insurance companies, too, don't see it that way. But I think that once the doctors see us as therapeutic and give orders for RT, the insurance companies will come around. Right now, we don't need an order to get patients involved in leisure services. There's really something to be able to charge for services because if you can bill, you're bringing in money and then you've got clout. We could hire some people—more RTs—and become what I see as a really professional service department....

I think the field is moving in the direction of leisure assessment more and more. And I think you'll see other things like the diagnosis of leisure problems and organized ways of treating the problems and ways to measure progress—the whole ball of wax. That's really where the limelight is, but there are real needs too. They're just going unnoticed and unconcerned. Let's face it. If what you're doing doesn't look like it fits within the medical model, you can just forget your credibility around here! As I said before, I think that part of the problem is the image of RT. It still has that activities-department-anyone-can-do-it image. Really!

All in all, as the director of leisure services states explicitly, the image of professional treatment emulates the medical model. Regardless of the specific service offered—whether OT, PT, speech, social services, leisure services, psychological consults, or nursing —the ideal image of professional treatment is one in which it is recognized that patients have extant, service-specific rehabilitation problems to which appropriate, credentialed judgment and expert treatment are applied in the best interest of the patient's rehabilitation, and which effect progress in rehabilitation in their own right.

The Image of Recovery

What is the image of treatment effectiveness in physical disability? Does treatment effect recovery or does "spontaneous" recovery allow for the effective application of treatment? It is not altogether clear whether recovery is due more to the application of medical or educational skills. The image of the place of treatment in recovery from physical disabilities—whether OT, PT, speech therapy, counseling, or leisure therapy—centers on this causal tension. While one image of Wilshire portrays it as a hospital, with its various services emulating a medical model, therapists of the services also speak of their treatment efforts as educational. The latter portrays recovery as a product of successful teaching and learning—for example, the successful teaching and learning of walking (gait training). The image of recovery is a tense mixture of medical success and guidance.

Consider the educational side of the image. One important educational goal is something called "muscle reeducation," which is the responsibility of the physical and occupational therapists. (Speech therapists also participate in reeducation but mainly in the area of cognition rather than musculature.) Like most teachers, the therapists believe that their students must possess certain traits, characteristics, or skills in order to take full advantage of training offered. Some of these, such as motivation or attitude, can be worked on during training sessions. Others, like sufficient intelligence, are not subject to modification. The most difficult aspect of readiness or preparedness for therapists is what they refer to as "return." For the most part, therapists do not explicitly claim that they actually can make nerves fire again or muscles flex and extend. Return of these functions is ostensibly a matter of the body gradually healing itself, but this is left largely unspecified. Once muscle function has returned, therapists work on strengthening and improving related skills such as balance and coordination.

"Readiness" is an important consideration for all patients. Therapists feel that the amputee should not be admitted to the hospital until the stump is healed sufficiently to permit exercise. Similarly, they feel that a person with a spinal injury must be emotionally prepared for physical therapy. The greatest challenge in assessing readiness, however, comes from persons who have suffered strokes or head trauma. They have multiple afflictions, in muscles, nerves, and cognitive processing; some will never have sufficient return of function to justify therapy, especially those patients with strokes or head injuries over a year old. In such cases, therapists see little chance for much more improvement. On the other hand, patients whose incidents are too recent are also not felt to be ready for rehab treatment. Therapists prefer to have some information from the acute care hospital indicating that the patient is medically stable and has some return of function before he is admitted to Wilshire. Whether treatment is portrayed as medical or educational, recovery is related to return of function.

The medical side of the image of recovery presents it as an achievement of therapeutic intervention: something the therapists do effects changes in the patient with physical disabilities. For example, as a result of his hospitalization, a paraplegic recovers adequately to be discharged to a relatively normal way of living; or a stroke victim who entered the hospital with right hemiplegia and aphasia is discharged with some mild paralysis in the right upper extremity and only slurred speech. In both instances hospital treatment is said to have effected considerable progress in recovery.

The tension between medical and educational interpretations of the process of recovery is apparent in the lingering doubts expressed by therapists about the causal mechanisms behind progress. There are well-known cases of patients who suddenly start walking one day after being totally unable to move their legs. Did such patients have need for exercise or muscle re-education? There are stories of persons who suddenly start to talk intelligibly after weeks of babbling and concomitant therapeutic effort. While more or less well-known, such cases are said to be the exception rather than the rule, the rule being an image of progress in recovery more or less resulting from therapeutic intervention, whether primarily medical or educational. The same ambiguity exists in interpretations of failure. The tension in images of recovery is only resolved in practice. Why and how a patient recovers from a physical disability may be portrayed as more or less the result of medical or educational intervention, depending on the particular audience.

Image of the Ideal Patient

A persistent theme in Wilshire talk about the behavior of patients in treatment is the importance of activity. While in the hospital, activity translates into "hard work" for patients under the direction of the therapists. It means attending therapy regularly, doing one's assigned exercises ("homework") in the evening and on weekends, and, more generally, assuming a serious stance toward rehabilitation by taking concerted advantage of the services offered. Staff members emphasize the "hard work" theme by contrasting Wilshire patients' behavior with that of patients in nursing homes or acute care hospitals. The ideal patient is foreseen as maximally independent after discharge. A person who does as much as possible toward recovery will feel better physically, have a more positive self-concept, and have better relations with others. Numerous stories are told of persons who made good progress while at Wilshire but who regressed after discharge because they let other people do things for them, things they could have done for themselves. Patients and their families are frequently warned about this. Even patients who will be almost totally dependent on others are to be taught to think of themselves as independent.

During treatment, staff members continually assess patients' activity levels and degrees of independence. Some patients are said to be capable of considerable independence but are "weak" and "susceptible" to the well-meant but harmful efforts of family members to assist them. Others are seen as "dependent personalities" or "institutional types" who feign dependence in order to get others to do things for them and also may be cleverly manipulative. A persistent byproduct of the emphasis on work and activity is staff members' fear that they may be unintentionally teaching dependent attitudes and habits through institutional living, where meals and some amount of personal care are provided and regular therapy is required. When this is seen as a clear possibility, some therapists recommend discharge, even though they believe further progress could be made at Wilshire. They feel that patients need to "get on the outside" and find out what independent living is all about.

As much as independent activity is valued as an ideal, however, it can go too far. Some patients are said to be "too independent," or "overresponsive." They may invent their own techniques for "doing transfers"—moving oneself from one location to another— or claim, say, that conversations with family or other patients is more important for their speech than what they do in speech therapy. While at times therapists approve of such independence and admit that patients can even teach them, at other times they describe the patient as "too stubborn" or as "not knowing what's good for him." One patient provided a particularly good example of how staff react to patients' assertiveness in pushing their own plans for therapy. The man was a diabetic who had had one leg amputated below the knee. Therapists and other staff members were trying to reduce the swelling in his stump and strengthen the leg so that he could begin working with a pylon (a temporary prothesis). He was doing his exercises regularly and the leg was unusually strong, but the swelling persisted, and he would have to stay longer than expected so that the problem could be corrected. Since the patient was anxious "to go home and resume my own life," this news upset him. He was particularly angry with the staff for their failure to reduce the swelling. He claimed this was due to the fact that they did not know how to regulate his insulin intake. He had been monitoring it for thirty years by himself and knew the proper balance, but claimed that the doctor and nurses at Wil- shire would not listen. As far as he was concerned, the only way he could get better was to get out of the hospital and learn to use the prosthesis on an outpatient basis. When he checked himself out of the hospital, the staff had mixed reactions. On the one hand, they were glad to be rid of a troublesome patient but, on the other, they were concerned about his condition and felt he did not know how to take care of himself properly; after all, they argued, if he had followed professional advice, he might never have lost the leg in the first place.

Patients said to be independent are those who speak of a strong desire to regain lost functions and to return to a way of life that, if not very similar in every way to their former life, is at least one where they can manage most things by themselves. Independent patients come to therapy on time, do what they are told, complete their homework in the evening, and express confidence in their progress. They do not criticize the therapist or the hospital, at least not much, nor do they invent their own therapies, at least as chal- lenges to programmed therapies. And they do not suggest that they really need to leave Wilshire so they can work at recovery on their own. While the image of the ideal patient is one that portrays him as hardworking and aiming for independent functioning, it is an image that separates the contexts of hard work and independence. While a patient is in therapy at Wilshire, he works hard (is "motivated") and aims for independence but does not display it in a manner contrary to therapeutic regimen. Patients are in the hospital, after all, to regain independence, not to declare it. Upon discharge the ideal patient is maximally independent.

The Course of Progress

While most everyone at the hospital agrees that the progress of patients toward independent living is their most general goal, images vary as to the typical course of progress. One set of images arises from the linear model in which progress unfolds in a step-like fashion, with small increments occurring with each day of therapy. Another set of images or model portrays progress as stage-like, wherein little or no change occurs for a period of time and then, at some critical point, the patient leaps to a new level (plateau) of recovery where gains must be consolidated before further progress can occur. There is also a "spontaneous" model wherein patients go from little or no progress to remarkable gains, perhaps approaching recovery, almost overnight. Staff members sometimes describe patients who "just popped out of it all of a sudden." Each set of images or model also allows for regression.

These images or models are articulated through interpretations of the individual patient's potential and other background information available to staff members. For example, physicians sometimes admit a person even though reports from an acute care hospital provide little reason to expect much progress. They do so because they see some "potential" in the patient. In this regard, one physician justified his decision by claiming, "I just saw some spark in there that made me hopeful." Staff sometimes recommend continued stay for a patient, beyond what past progress might ordinarily justify, because of "potential." The argument for "potential" is linked with ideas about the recovery-effectiveness of motivation, supportive families, a good sense of humor, a strong desire to live independently, among other telling background characteristics. Those patients who possess a good share of these attributes are seen as having good potential for making progress and as being good candidates for rehabilitation. Thus staff members can "read" the typical potential of individual patients and assign it a course of progress.

Chapter 3

Working with the Patient

Staff members do not speak to patients in the same way they talk or report to families and third parties, even though the common topic of their communications is physical rehabilitation. Some of this difference results from the varying kinds of information sought by the different people involved with the patient's rehabilitation. For example, a young wife might ask Wilshire therapists how to exercise her husband's partially paralyzed legs when he returns home, while his insurance company might ask them to provide detailed information about what specific treatments they have prescribed for him and why.

But there is another variation in staff members' descriptions. Staff members, more or less wittingly, consider their audience's concerns and frames of reference. Whether members of different audiences raise similar or dissimilar substantive questions about, say, treatment effectiveness, the staff members will frame their answers in terms of what they assume to be concerns relevant to the audiences. They will articulate their descriptions against a background of beliefs about what certain audiences do, or should, think about the specific realities of physical rehabilitation.

How does the therapist incorporate images of place and treatment in communications with the working patient? In this chapter we consider the working patient as an audience for the therapist's description and conversation about treatment and response.

IMAGES AND THE WORKING PATIENT

An ideal patient is an appropriate admission. That is, he needs some form of rehabilitative treatment—chiefly physical therapy—has potential for improvement, and strives for independence. He is a medically stable patient who may safely leave the care of nurse and physician to undergo rehabilitative treatment. A patient who suffers from, say, chronic diarrhea or who contracts influenza is considered unfit for physical rehabilitation or, if not unfit, difficult to accommodate in intensive regimens of therapy. The ideal patient is also mentally alert enough to understand directions and respond to them intelligibly.

The working patient is the particular person literally *embodying* the dysfunction encountered by clinical staff. The working patient may not approach the "ideal" patient but, at the very least, is understandable in terms of the standard. He or she may or may not need physical rehabilitation, for merely having a dysfunction, such as right hemiplegia, is not necessarily an indication for rehabilitation therapy. In addition, a patient suffering from an "old stroke"—a stroke that occurred over one year before hospital admission—has functional inadequacies and thus a need for rehabilitation, but no potential for recovery.

Old strokes are the most common cases of need without potential. The patient tends to be middle-aged or older, as are most stroke victims. He or she may have been briefly hospitalized in an acute care facility immediately following the stroke. When the patient's condition became medically stable, he or she might have been discharged to an extended-care or skilled nursing facility, a nursing home. Such a patient may languish in an unchanged condition in the nursing home and, several months or a year later, be transferred to Wilshire at the behest of a family who desires or detects improvement.

One rule-of-thumb for distinguishing between patients with recovery potential and those without is to determine the length of time that has passed since the onset of the condition leading to physical dysfunction. Such a determination is condition-specific. In the case of stroke victims, the time criterion is one year. In other cases, the time is less explicit but still a workable criterion.

Using the rule-of-thumb is not a straightforward matter; therapists interpret the applicability of the time criterion case by case, justifying their decisions accordingly. An elderly female stroke victim who is encountered by a therapist fifteen months after her accident, and who regains no functions two weeks after intensive therapy at Wilshire, is said to be "an old stroke, after all" and not a good candidate for continued hospitalization. The same therapist may encounter another elderly female with the very same fifteen-month-old condition and yet not label her an old stroke when she shows no improvement after several weeks in therapy. Why this discrepancy in prognoses? In the latter case the therapist is informed by a social worker that the patient spent a year in a nursing home but "wasn't even given a chance to improve because they [nursing home staff] kept her in bed all the time." The patient is thus taken to be an exception to the one-year rule. The therapist concludes, "She's not really an old stroke, you see." Rather, she is considered to be the typical stroke patient who has potential for improvement. The former patient, in contrast, is considered a "typical" old stroke.

Whether there is validity to such differentiations on objective grounds may enter into different interpretations of patients' typical status. Although objective grounds do not, in their own right, form the basis of these different determinations regarding patient status, they are used to support or discredit the determination. For example, when confronted with the discrepancy in the status of the two stroke patients, a therapist stated that she "knows for a fact" and "what's more, it's common knowledge" that the nursing home from which the "real" old stroke was transferred to Wilshire "has a very good PT department" and that the facility from which the other patient was discharged has "not much to speak of, really."

There is no particular time at which patients are judged conclusively to be in need of, or as having potential for, rehabilitation. Such judgments can be made at any point in the course of the patient's hospitalization. A year-old stroke, for example, may have been admitted to Wilshire with "great potential," for reasons similar to those just discussed, but be recommended for discharge four weeks later when it is realized that the patient had been a "typical" old stroke all along, for some reason or other that was not known earlier.

Whether or not the patient approaches the ideal in terms of need and potential for rehabilitation, staff members' beliefs about what needs and potential are typical serve as the working frame from which they organize their interaction with them. A patient who, at some point, is considered to have no potential is treated by the therapists rather unenthusiastically. As a speech therapist put it:

Oh sure. You continue to see the patient but you more or less just go through the motions until he or she is discharged. What else can you do? Somewhere along the line, someone—me or someone else—was wrong about this particular patient. That's all.

Beliefs and decisions about potential are validated by, and confirm, the staff's approach to the patient in treatment. Once a therapist sees that a patient is an old stroke, a perfunctory course of interaction seems reasonable, given the assessment of the patient's "typical" status. In turn, the ongoing course of interaction serves to confirm the belief in the patient's hopeless lack of potential. Accordingly, the therapist may explain, for example, "Of course, there's not much potential. Just look at what we do day after day... not much of anything."

The manner in which staff members relate to patients and describe their treatment, how they attempt to control patients' responses to treatment (encouraging or discouraging them), and the reasons they provide for progress or the lack thereof, are informed largely and deliberately by an educational image of place and treatment. Therapists' working concern with rehab potential is a hallmark of the image, centering importantly on the issue of whether there is potential for learning. Staff members act toward patients as teachers toward students. They are prepared to teach patients with potential how to regain normal or maximal functioning and to prepare them to lead as near to independent lives as possible. They orient themselves to think of the patient as someone who has more or less potential for learning—a potential affected by medical, cognitive, and motivational factors. To this end, they refer to the hospital in various ways as an educational institution. While a medical orientation has a place in therapists' work with patients, it is part of an image of rehabilitation understood as more uniformly relevant to families and third parties.

When therapists encounter new patients, they introduce themselves and exchange information with the patients about their backgrounds and sentiments about any number of current events in and out of the hospital, among other topics of casual conversation. Therapists say that they try to "get to know each patient as a person" before they begin assessment and treatment. Considerable give-and-take occurs in the exchanges, much of which is initially aimed at locating some common ground. A therapist asks patients about their families, parents, or children, where they work or worked before retirement, where they live. Should a patient, for example, state that he was a supervisor at a local manufacturing plant for thirty years before he retired, his therapist might remark, "My father worked in that plant, too!", whereupon both patient and therapist attempt to trace further ties based on this common feature of their backgrounds.

Common ground is not fully established, once and for all, on first encounters. It unfolds as therapist and patient interact daily throughout the course of the patient's hospitalization and serves to integrate the lives within the institution. Both therapist and patient experience the integration in casual and working conversations. For example, in the second week of therapy, the aforementioned therapist may greet the patient with, "Hi, Mr. American Motors!", to which the patient responds jokingly, "You better take it easy on us American Motors people. Your dad wouldn't want you beating up on him like you beat up on me yesterday." Recognition of their common background serves as a means to strengthen their interpersonal bond and the special mutual obligations that may be expected to result from it. To have common ground is to have a referential means of influence. Either patient or therapist can describe and prescribe his or her actions in relation to common grounds and, thereby, shape the ongoing interaction.

Other background information, not necessarily common, is also shared. While the information does not tie therapist and patient to each other in the same way a common background does, other information also generates a mutually recognizable context for describing and discussing treatment and responses to treatment. Thus, while a patient may have no connection with the particular prestigious school which the therapist at one time mentioned attending, the patient can use the information in the therapeutic situation by, for example, mentioning (and thereby suggesting) when the therapist grows impatient because the patient can't do as well as the therapist expected, to slow down because "I didn't have all that fancy schooling you got and I have to think things out."

Both therapist and patient use background information—that which they have in common as well as that which they do not—to describe their activities and their ongoing, desirable, and undesirable features. As soon as therapist and patient encounter each other, they begin to build an interpersonal basis for verbally informing and influencing each other. As therapy progresses, another kind of context begins to emerge from the history of their therapeutic interaction: its trials, triumphs, casual talk, amusements, disappointments. This, together with background information, serves both patient and therapist as a resource that influences the shape of their relationship as student and teacher.

Background information shared by patient and therapist thus affects assessment and treatment, not as superficial chitchat carried on in connection with them, but as an integral feature of accomplishing them. Relating to the patient as teacher to student, the therapist uses background information in teaching how to regain useful functioning. The physical therapist, for example, does not simply manipulate the patient's lower extremities. She also describes, say, how the patient is or is not walking. In attempts to obtain a correct response, the therapist calls upon accumulated knowledge about the patient to explain why the patient can do better, should not go faster, why the therapist could not do as well, among many other means of influencing the patient to do one thing or another. For example, with the knowledge that both the therapist's own father and the patient were American Motors employees (the common recognition that the therapist's father and the patient are alike in this regard), the therapist urges the lackadaisical patient to put more effort into the ranging exercises because "I know *my* father would have really put all *he* had into it."

The therapist "knows" that her skills in relation to the working patient are aimed at getting the patient to respond in kind, but independently, to what she demonstrates through body movements and instructional skill. The physical therapist, for instance, walks down the hall and describes each move to show the patient how to walk. The speech therapist sounds words out and explains how she physically produced the sounds. The social worker and leisure therapist counsel the patient by explaining, for example, how to be more assertive or how to plan a useful future. Whatever is taught, the therapist expects that demonstration of a functional skill will be followed by the patient's attempt to do likewise: the teacher demonstrates how; the student tries to emulate by applying the knowledge and rules the teacher has supplied. Given the need and the potential for rehabilitation, the working patient is shown how to improve. Like a student, the patient is expected to apply what has been taught. An occupational therapist, for example, might show a patient how to adapt arthritic hands to the detailed demands of embroidery and then assign several stitches to the patient for homework, to be completed later that day and before the OT session the next morning.

Therapists use educational terminology in describing their own and the patient's therapeutic activity. Key terms reference the image. Therapists constantly tell patients what they are going to *teach* them. They inform patients that they must *practice* in order to *learn* what they have been taught. They give them *homework* and later ask patients if they completed their *assignments*. When patients fail to do their homework or the therapist determines that the patient is "getting by too easy," the patient may be given *extra homework*. It is not unusual for the therapist to refer to the patient explicitly as a good, poor, improving, well-motivated, or some such *student*. And likewise, patients occasionally refer to their therapists as *teachers*, some good, some demanding, and so on. Whether the working patient learns slowly or rapidly, is moderately or strongly motivated, he nonetheless is considered to be and to respond to therapists like a student. The conception of Wilshire as a school, the image of place, informs the image of patients as students and the expectation of therapists that they will respond as such. The working patient enters, learns or does not learn at a particular pace, and is promoted or discharged to his or her future.

Should the patient become medically unstable, should he or she be virtually incommunicable, have no potential, or be completely lacking in interest in rehabilitation, other images suggest themselves to, and are referenced by, therapists. When the patient contracts a real or alleged medical problem, when he or she remains indisposed over several days, not attending therapies, it may be suggested that he or she be discharged until the capacity for physical rehabilitation is regained. Such patients are told that they must either attend their therapies or recuperate elsewhere. One patient, for example, who convalesced alone for a week in her room and the following week participated quite unenthusiastically in her therapy, while complaining about her aches and pains, was told pointedly by her occupational therapist, "You're just going to have to be transferred to St. Catherine's [an acute care hospital] or somewhere else to get better if you're not going to try to put in some effort here to do what we're trying to teach you."

When, however, the patient is so aphasic as to be virtually incommunicable, therapists find it difficult to teach. They try various means of reaching such patients, many of whom are stroke victims. They may resort to an improvised sign language; modalities like writing are attempted; sometimes a communication board works. For some aphasic patients, nothing seems to get through. On occasion, a therapist will be overloaded with such patients. Because therapists often say that they prefer to have a variety of patients—some strokes, some spinal cord injured, arthritics, a few amputees—at such times they report that they may feel they are working in a nursing home rather than in a rehab hospital.

On occasion a therapist encounters a patient who is medically fit to participate in therapy, who is alert, but who has little or no interest in therapy. Such patients may scoff at the therapist's efforts and the various treatment programs in general but make no effort to be discharged. These patients, who make use of the hospital's bed-and-board facilities while resisting treatment, are said to be using the hospital like a hotel. There may be no place to discharge them readily. A patient seen in this way by a therapist may be reminded, in subtle or direct terms, that Wilshire is neither a sanitarium nor a spa and that the therapists and clinical staff are not just around to wait on them.

While the image of the working patient held by all staff members may vary from being educational to medical, convalescent, or recreational, all staff are prepared to act educationally when dealing with the patient therapeutically. They see and articulate their skills in a pedagogical manner and they depend on the patient to respond in a like manner. Indeed, they understand their success in these terms. While staff know in various ways that in order for them to teach and for the student to put what he or she has been taught into effect, the patient must have some physical potential for learning, progress is described by staff to the patient in terms of what both do to impede or enhance learning. In relation to the working patient, progress in rehabilitation is primarily a matter of good teaching and eager learning rather than "return of function."

PRESENTING THE IMAGE

Initial encounters with new patients are mainly informational. Two kinds of information are exchanged. One is an exchange of background information, discussed briefly in the last section: introductions take place and the therapist asks questions about the patient's background; in turn, information about the therapist's background is offered. The background information, common or otherwise, now serves and will continue to serve as means of making relevant the various ongoing actions of both patient and therapist in treatment. A second kind of information exchanged in initial encounters concerns treatment prospects. An occupational therapist, for example, informs a patient that he is scheduled for thirty minutes of OT daily and describes what will occur in that time. The therapist informs the patient about what the therapist, will be doing and what is expected from the patient in return. The information exchanged revolves around how each of them will participate in therapy and what might best be their common orientation for the most beneficial results. The therapist thus begins to teach the patient about their respective therapy roles.

Consider the following excerpt from a conversation between a female occupational therapist and a twenty-three-year-old male paraplegic at their initial encounter. She interviews him in his room on one of the nursing units. As therapists frequently note, some patients either do not believe that much of anything can be done for them or they think that the hospital is there to cure them in some way. The first problem is one of poor motivation; the second is one of inappropriate image. The therapist tries to deal with the problems immediately, lest her prospective pupil have the wrong idea of what is forthcoming.

[*The therapist (OT) enters the patient's (Pt) room and finds him in his wheelchair watching a portable television set.*]

OT: Hi. How are you today?

Pt: I'm okay, I guess. Who're you?

OT: I'm Linda Stephens and I'm your occupational therapist. You'll be working with me in OT. Right now I think we've got you scheduled for 10 o'clock in the morning. We might increase that later depending on how you do. Okay?

Pt: Okay.

OT: I'd like to tell you a little about what we're going to be doing, okay? One of the main things we do in OT is called "power-building." We want to get those arms working up to their highest potential. You're going to be using your arms a lot, a lot more than they've ever been used before.

Pt: There's nothing wrong with my arms. It's these legs. They don't move...and they're not going to ever move. Right? [*Therapist doesn't answer.*] So...so what can you do about it? I mean there's not much that anyone can do about it. Right? Right! I'm really not sure why I'm here anyway. First the doctor tells me that...I'm going to be a cripple for the rest of my life. So he hit me with that. That's like being hit by a Mack truck and....

OT: I understand you were in a car accident.

[*Patient describes the car accident in some detail. He then relates his previous hospital experiences, what he was told about spinal cord injuries of his type, and how he felt during recovery. The occupational therapist sympathizes.*]

OT: That's a normal kind of reaction. It's not uncommon. I know how you feel. After all, it means a change in your whole way of life...but it doesn't mean that you have to give up on life, you know. You're a young guy and have great potential. And we're here to help you make something of it.

Pt: [*Sighs*] Oh, I don't know....

OT: Now look. That's no attitude to take. I've seen many guys with much worse injuries pick themselves up by the bootstraps and really get it together. What did you do before your accident?

[*Patient describes his job, where he lived, and tells the therapist about his family. She shares with him similar background information about herself. They have a few things in common, which both eagerly pursue with interest and surprise. There is much more they do not share in common. The therapist then returns to her description of OT.*]

OT: Well, okay, now let me tell you what we'll be doing. Besides the powerbuilding stuff I told you about, we'll get involved in home-making skills. That's when we teach you about different ways to get around your apartment. They're a lot of neat things to help you make cleaning up and cooking and getting around easier....

[*Therapist elaborates. Patient responds unenthusiastically.*]

Pt: I guess so...oh I don't know. I'm here, but what for? You know what I mean? It can't be cured. That's what they told me. So what am I doing here in the hospital again. Huh?

OT: Look, you just remember; you're here to learn. Just keep thinking that. You understand? You're just going to have to get that cure stuff out of your head. I mean it's not going to get you anywhere. You're only going to do as well as what *you, you* put into it. We're here to teach you how to adapt to your disability. If you're ready to learn, you'll learn a lot. I know. I've seen it. Look, no one is going to wave a magic wand over you and, zap, and you're going to walk out of here. A guy with your background...just look at all those things you've accomplished all on your own. You can't tell me all of that is gone. If you take advantage of this place, you'll see.

Pt: Yeah, I know.

OT: Okay, then. Let's have a more positive attitude about it. I'll see you tomorrow in the OT clinic. That's right down the hall to your left. One of the runners [escort aides] will pick you up just before 10. You be ready, okay?

Not all patients are poorly motivated nor do they all have what therapists consider to be an inappropriate image of treatment, such as a disgruntled expectation to be cured. Some come into the hospital ready and eager to begin their programs; some are too eager, referred to by therapists as "overresponsiveness," which is considered to be a motivational and patient management problem. Some also enter Wilshire with a rather precise image of how the therapist expects to see the working patient. However, except for clues gleaned by therapists from family members about prospective patients in this regard, or from other staff members (what a social worker, for example, may pass on to OT about the patient based on an intake interview), or from incoming records, it is not known "what the patient will actually be like" as a prospective student. Regardless of what turns out to be the case and whether that changes several times in the course of hospitalization, therapists use their initial encounters with patients to, in effect, set the scene and present the actors: to inform the patients of what they will be doing, to teach them the expected attitude—the role they each will be expected to play in therapy—and the probable outcome of having done all of this well.

The working patient is primarily someone whose effort and learning skill the rehabilitation therapist will depend on for progress. A number of therapists report that they only become fully aware of the significance and importance of this on the job. One therapist (OT) reported that her formal training primarily stressed, as she put it, the "body, muscles, and anatomy stuff," which she contrasted with what she called "the real world."

> I know when I first came to work here, when I first got out of OT, I soon found out that what I learned at school is one thing and what you do on the job is another thing. Here you're in the real world. When you're here, you have to work with patients, not just muscles and bodies. There [at school] they feed you all that body, muscles, and anatomy stuff. And, of course, you get to know all that...but we're not really doing body stuff, I mean in the same way. We're trying to get these people to get their acts together. You just have to get after some of them. And some do and some don't. But you just never know until you get to know each one. And, like I said, they don't teach you much about that in school.

While the educational image is the one preferred by therapists for organizing their descriptive encounters with working patients, the limitations of the skills that foster this image is also critically assessed by therapists themselves. Whether in speech, OT, PT, leisure services, or social work, therapists contrast the kind of professional training they received with the ongoing character of their work with rehab patients.

Many therapists see their professional training as patterned after a medical model of treatment in which they learn that patients have problems, that problems are treatable, and that the effective application of treatment normalizes functioning. Their training consequently centers on learning two kinds of knowledge. One focuses on service-specific conditions; speech therapists for example, take speech pathology courses in which they learn about the mechanisms of normal and pathological speech and oral anatomy, and physical therapists learn about human musculature and anatomy. The second kind of knowledge focuses on service-specific assessment and treatment strategies. For example, speech therapists learn how to administer the Porch Index of Communicative Ability (PICA) and the Minnesota Test for Differential Diagnosis of Aphasia. Leisure or recreation therapists become proficient in administering leisure attitude scales. All therapists learn about a range of treatment strategies applicable to problems in their respective areas: OTs learn about energy conservation techniques and safety skills; social workers are taught techniques of crisis intervention; physical therapists learn that special modalities, such as hydrotherapeutic apparatus and diathermy, are available to treat patients' dysfunctions. But despite all of this, their training is organized around a conception of what they will do which glosses over the interactive complexity of their relationship with patients, something which therapists partially frame in educational terms.

While therapists sometimes complain about how impractical their skills are when encountering the working patient, they are not necessarily dissatisfied with what they know nor with the skills they possess. When they arise, complaints concern lack of formal skill in modulating and articulating medically oriented training with interactive contingencies. Periodic vexation sometimes leads them to raise questions about what their own and their patients' roles are in therapy—questions of how they present themselves to each other in practice—as therapist/patient or as teacher/student? The former image suggests that what therapists do directly alters dysfunction. The latter image suggests that what therapists inform patients about, demonstrate to them, and convince them to realize on their own alters dysfunction. Therapists sometimes feel unprepared to deal with the working patient but they are not dissatisfied, on the whole, with what they know technically about patient problems and how to assess and treat them.

The distinction between the therapist/patient and the teacher/student relationship is both explicit and vague. There are occasions when the distinction is recognized openly. For example, in the PT office doing "paper work" before, between, and after scheduled therapies, physical therapists sometimes talk about or debate the issue of what, as they say, "we're actually doing for patients any-

way." Looking over a patient's recorded progress, a therapist comments casually, "This is really the pits. I ask myself what am I
really doing with Tom and the others. Even if I do everything just
so-so and work my tail off, can I say I'm really getting through to
him?" Thereupon, various therapists—some more and some less
explicitly—speak of and comment on what precisely their roles
are in actually working with patients, about whether they're really
"just here to coach these people along," or whether they can "really
do something" to effect rehabilitation.

This issue is directly broached while working with patients. As
the OT (whose initial encounter with her 23-year-old patient was
excerpted) warned the patient, "You should get that cure stuff out
of your head." She went on to describe an alternate relationship,
one in which she would not attempt to cure the patient of his dysfunction but teach him about his problem and how *he* might adapt
to it. The issue is again raised directly in ongoing therapy. On one
occasion, an occupational therapist who had grown increasingly
frustrated that an arthritic patient's disinterest in the therapist's
attempt to demonstrate how to make use of the functioning re-
maining in the patient's hands, explained: "Look, my friend, all I
can do is show you and encourage you. The rest is up to you. There's
no way I can make your problem go away. Let's just face it. I don't
have a bag of tricks. C'mon, let's put more into this, okay?"

At other times the distinction made between the two role relationships is rather vague. Ongoing conversations between therapists
about patients and between individual working patients and their
therapists confound the medical and educational images of the
relationship. A patient may refer to what is occurring in treatment
as the result of having such a skilled therapist, whereupon the
therapist maintains that the patient is being taught how to function properly and that any progress is due to the patient's willingness to learn. On the other hand, a patient who repeatedly scoffs
at the therapist's efforts may be reminded that the patient is there
to be rehabilitated by highly skilled people, not to play games.

Conversations between therapists indicate that they, too, confound the distinction between the medical and educational images
of rehab roles. One therapist may boast to another that "I really
brought Sharon around in the last week"—that treatment efforts
had effected progress. A second therapist responds, "That's great,
isn't it? You really can see a difference when they get some return
and get it together." As the conversation unfolds, both therapists
gloss over the issue of whether they understood each other—
whether the therapist effected progress or whether the joint efforts

of patient and therapist coincided with a return of function. Regardless of what actually occurred, one therapist takes pride in particular efforts expended, and the other compliments the "therapist's" achievement. How the achievement came about, and to what extent it was a joint activity, was not clear.

Teaching Roles

Whether fully recognized or not, therapists speak of their roles as teachers in different ways; they do not all perceive their teaching activity similarly. In addition, the meaning of being a student and learning also varies. At one extreme is the therapist who sees the therapeutic role as "didactic," as one social worker put it. This teaching role emphasizes the active guidance of teaching functional skills to rehab patients. It is active in the sense that the teaching function is seen as pivotal in the recovery of the patient, and the key to progress lies in the active intervention of the therapist in particular rehab problems. It is therefore not so much the patient who effects progress alone as the therapist who intervenes and thereby organizes the patient's motivation along an effective course for recovery. In this way active intervention is guided: the didactic therapist not only presses the patient toward progress but organizes it along lines considered both individually and clinically suitable.

The didactic orientation to teaching may, of course, like any orientation, run up against an unmotivated patient, one who is not too enthusiastic about prospects for recovery, one who presents lack of enthusiasm in lethargic responses to the therapist's efforts and in erratic attendance at scheduled therapy sessions. A didactic teacher aggressively attempts to build the patient's motivation, to make a good student out of him, to "whip up his enthusiasm," as a leisure therapist asserted. On that basis, the therapist guides the patient to recovery.

The didactic therapist "knows" what is best for the patient. While relying on the patient to be a good student, an eager learner, the therapist knows that it is he or she who holds the key to progress; training and experience have provided answers that the patient does not have. At best, the "good" patient "catches on" and emulates what has been taught.

While the didactic therapist sees all efforts to guide and motivate as directed at the patient's improvement, it would be a mistake to consider the didactic therapist haughty about treatment. On the contrary, the therapist's understanding of this role is one that, in its articulation, "can make a difference in the patient's recovery and future lifestyle." In complaining to a social worker about one of their mutual patients, a speech therapist made this very point:

Hey, Toots, I'm no wallflower around here. That guy [patient] thinks he's going to walk right out of here and go back to school and graduate next summer. No way! Yeah, he wants to get better. Sure! But he doesn't know what he's talking about. Literally! *I know* what's best for the guy and I work myself to the bone trying to get him to improve his grammar and speech. He's always saying I'm lording it over him. Boy, is he on the wrong track. Sweetheart, he just don't know. That's all. And I do. I wish you'd talk to him, for his own good.

The didactic therapist speaks of the relationship with the patient and presents an attitude focused on what the therapist can do for the patient "for his or her own good," if the patient cooperates. Indeed, the phrase "for [the patient's] own good" is shorthand for this orientation to teaching; it is an index of the didactic image. What is taught is for the patient's good; but the therapist, not the patient, defines the good. Because the therapist, not the patient, knows what the patient's future will be like if progress is not made in rehabilitation, this knowledge informs the therapist that, for the patient's own good, it is the therapist who can make a difference. The therapist's job is therefore to get the patient to build a better future, a future that can be more satisfying than the one currently facing him. Like the adage about the teacher who molds minds and shapes young lives, the didactic therapist builds futures.

Standing in contrast to the didactic view of the therapeutic role is an orientation that one social worker described as that of "facilitator." The social worker commented on this image of rehabilitation, as opposed to the more didactic orientation, just after completing what was portrayed as a frustrating family conference. It was apparent that some of the staff were "pretty didactic," while others, like the speaker, saw themselves as facilitators. The two orientations clashed in presenting the patient's course of treatment to family members.

I know that many of the staff feel that they're teaching the clients. They have a didactic orientation. They want to teach the client all kinds of things that he really knows how to do himself. I mean any reasonable person would and could do what the therapists and the social workers feel they have to teach them. I just don't see it that way. I see myself as more of a facilitator, as someone who gets patients to help themselves and each other. Of course, I'm not the only one. There are a few OTs and some PTs who feel the same way. It's really a different point of view on what we're here for and what we're supposed to be doing.

I'd like to set up something like self-help groups where patients can learn from each other and can help each other to solve their problems, directly related...or indirectly related...to their particular handicaps. And I don't mean like Sam Burton's [a consulting psychologist] spinal cord support group. That's all teaching...I mean that's okay too. I guess it's alright to be informed about all those facts about community services available to the handicapped. That's not what I have in mind. I mean a real self-help group, by and for those who know best the whats and whys of their problems.

The facilitator orientation to teaching is not considered one of active guidance. Rather, the facilitator provides the means for patients to teach themselves, to build their own futures. The facilitator asks the patients to explore their own future and to evaluate what the hospital, its staff members, and similarly handicapped patients can do to facilitate the individual patients' developing conception of what they hope to be and how they hope to live. The facilitator does not choose a course of treatment for the patients' own good, but presents them with alternatives. Such a therapist induces the patients to consider alternatives, both those described by the therapist and those discovered individually or by patients together. One occupational therapist, describing the teaching role in this way, remarked, "It's the patients' right. They have a right to participate directly in planning and deciding what we're going to work on. It's not my right to run the whole show." What to a didactic orientation is "for their own good," to a facilitating orientation is a matter of "patients' rights."

A good deal of piety is evidenced in the expression and presentation of both points of view. At times didactic therapists decry the fact that certain patients do not avail themselves of whatever therapeutic program is designed for them by the staff, programs that "we all know are for the patient's own good." At times facilitators say that they are irritated by patients who do not exercise their rights and actively contribute to their own rehabilitation. Like the didactic therapist, the facilitator also believes that he or she knows best.

The facilitator's concern with the patient's motivation is cast differently than that of the didactic therapist. The facilitator practices the role by "inviting" the patient to, at the very least, take the opportunity to consider his future and decide, in a rational and open fashion, between available alternatives. For example, the occupational therapist invites the patient to consider the kinds of skills necessary to live in a personally satisfying manner. Having discussed this with the patient, the therapist organizes the therapeutic program accordingly. In similar fashion, the physical therapist learns of the patient's future homemaking plans and attempts to schedule the treatment/teaching program around them. For example, if a spinal-cord injured patient plans to get around town in a modified van, the facilitating therapist suggests various exercises to enhance the realization of that patient's goal, such as working on "transfers" (moving one's body from place to place by sliding down a lightweight, portable board) or "wheelies" (balancing and manipulating a wheelchair up, down, and around curbs or other obstacles). The facilitator's view of futures is that, in general, the patient knows what's best in his or her particular case, and that he or she is reasonable enough to decide what is most suitable among the alternatives presented by the therapist and the hospital.

While in the final analysis both didactic and facilitative therapists may actually teach the same things to patients, the difference in their roles comes with how they present treatment to patients. The difference is practical in the sense that how a therapist presents herself or himself, and how this role presentation is seen by others, including patients and staff, is articulated within the ongoing working conditions of physical rehabilitation. In working with one patient, for example, an occupational therapist may present as a facilitator but, in working with another, may be more didactic. The difference between didactic and facilitating therapists is not one of character. To portray an individual therapist as, say, didactic, does not necessarily find that therapist organizing treatment of all patients in a didactic fashion. In the ongoing working affairs of clinical relations with patients, we do not find this kind of consistency. Rather, the difference is one in the practical presentation of teaching roles. On first encounter an individual therapist may present to a patient as a facilitator (whether explicitly or by inference). Later, we may find the therapist speaking to the same patient in a didactic fashion, even referring to what "is best" for the patient's "own good," pointing out that if the patient expects to make any significant improvement, attention might well best be paid to the therapeutic course that has been planned. On a still later occasion we hear that same therapist speak to the patient as one who provides patients with alternatives, with choices for developing futures, and of how both of them, together, can lay out a course of teaching and learning that "could make a difference." In practice, the individual therapist, as a teacher, is both didactic and facilitating.

The lack of consistency is not a sign of arbitrariness. If one's teaching orientation were simply a matter of character, this might be true. But, in practice, orientations are not organized in this way. From one circumstance to another, the therapist faces the working patient, day in and day out, as a particular person at a particular time, with current relevant desires, enthusiasm, and mood in relation to a particular life history and background. The therapist's conduct in the course of rehab work is organized to deal with specific conditions in the service of completing daily programs of treatment. It is these ongoing, circumstantial "projects" that therapists face in relation to the working patient, not a transcendent principle of consistency. Should consistency become a matter of principle for a therapist, it is an issue encountered and dealt with contextually, *within* the ongoing, specific activities with, or in relation to, patients.

Therapists do not so much identify the particular roles and expect patients to do likewise as they use particular teaching and learning roles to accomplish or interpret treatment and rehabilitation. Indeed, they use their varied notions of teaching and learning to explain their respective working identities. On occasion, therapists may explicitly and literally speak of themselves as "using what you have to," "doing what works best," and so forth. On other occasions, however, the orientations are spoken of implicitly and passively.

What appears to be settled, for practical purposes, on first encounters with patients is in fact continually subject to interpretation, refinement, and reinterpretation in the course of clinical activities. The presentation of roles becomes a practical *modus operandi* articulated within the ongoing, specific circumstances of work. Images of rehabilitation and orientations to treatment are the stock of available interpretations of clinical activities and therapeutic roles which the therapist uses to make sense of and to effect treatment and rehabilitation.

DOING THERAPY

Therapists more or less "know" that they are teachers and that progress depends significantly on whether the patient is a good student, but in order to enter into particular events and situations, the knowledge must be specified in terms of those situations. The concrete meaning of teaching on one occasion may or may not be identical with what it is on another occasion because the realities considered to be at stake in each are not necessarily the same. While the image of rehabilitation that serves as a background to relations with the working patient is largely educational, both therapists and working patients are continually active in interpreting images as a whole and their details in particular in concrete situations.

Consider how an educational image is articulated in relation to the working patient. While the content of therapy, say, in OT differs from leisure therapy and PT in terms of treatment technology, they are similar in how therapists describe and explain conduct, in how roles enter into what therapists do in relation to the working patient, and in the image is used to specify what is or what should be going on in therapy.

Specifying Standards

In the formal and informal organization of their teaching activity, therapists accept established, and specify particular, standards by which to judge the success of patients' responses to their efforts. Each discipline has available a variety of established standards for judging progress in rehabilitation. For example, in doing a series of exercises to develop the written communication skill of a stroke patient, a speech therapist makes use of a section of the "Language Rehabilitation Program," a therapeutic package used in rehab and other treatment facilities. The section consists of a series of picture cards, the relational contents of which the patient is asked to describe succinctly in one written sentence. On the back of each card is a suggested sentence describing the relationship of the card's pictured contents. The suggested sentences are the basis upon which the therapist assesses the student's progress in written communication skill. This exercise enables use of an established standard in making the assessment.

Therapists also specify additional standards for evaluating progress. They assess each patient's potential, motivation, background, possible future, and then set goals for rehabilitation. Some are general and unspecified while others are written up and become part of the patient's record. Some standards are informal and enter into the therapist's judgment of progress from day to day as working goals.

Whether established or specified, standards provide the therapist with a means of describing to the patient how well he or she is doing. For example, given that a physical therapist has informed a patient that the next lesson to be taught will be how to do bed transfers, the patient is instructed in how to use a transfer board efficiently to move between the wheelchair and bed. As instruction proceeds and the patient responds by trying out what has been demonstrated and explained, the therapist refers to the patient's success or lack of success in terms of what a successful bed transfer should be: the therapist describes the patient's efforts and what has been learned in terms of the standard.

The idea of a standard, established or not, is that it has some stability over the course of treatment. It need not be completely the same throughout but, at the very least, it should not change or be changed every time it is used to judge progress. It is a standard precisely because it does not change each time it is used.

The practice of judging the patient's progress shows, however, that the matter of deciding whether and how well a patient has learned is not a straightforward matter of comparing standards with patients' responses. In practice, therapists and patients interpret what the meaning of the standard is and what the meaning of their teaching and learning is each time judgments are made. Their interpretive activity literally gives concrete meaning to standards and patient progress. Indeed, concrete meaning must be given in order to make standards immediately sensible in ongoing rehabilitative practice.

Let us examine the practice of standard specification as a speech therapist makes use of parts of the Language Rehabilitation Program to improve written communication. The patient, Sharon, is a 28-year-old female who has suffered a stroke that initially left her unable to talk and barely walk. Since her accident, she has had considerable return of function. She now can talk, but haltingly and with slurred articulation. She is partially paralyzed on the right side, extensively in her right arm, which she carries in a sling. The speech therapist, Nancy, has placed a series of cards on the table in front of the patient and instructed her to write out one-sentence descriptions that relate the various objects depicted. The following conversation unfolds.

[*For a picture card depicting a girl and a tree, the patient has written "The tree is next to the girl."*]

Nancy: Well...I don't think so, Sharon. Now what could you do? How could you change that to make it more acceptable?

[*Sharon looks at the sentence and repeats it, not understanding her mistake.*]

Nancy: Look at it again. The way you have it written, it sounds like the tree is moving...sounds like the *tree* is standing next to the girl.

Sharon: Oh. [*Pause*] How about "The girl is standing next to the tree?"

Nancy: Yes. That's better.

The therapist has directed the patient's response so it comes closer to what is written on the back of the picture card. But what "more acceptable" means was not obvious in the therapist's initial instructions. Sharon understood her instructions to be to write single sentences relating the pictured objects. What the particular relationship should have been was left unspecified; the standard for being correct emerged only after Sharon wrote a sentence. Apparently what the therapist had in mind, but did not inform Sharon of, was that the relationship depicted should be active, in which one object is depicted as doing something to another rather than merely being juxtaposed. The therapist had available to her an established standard: the suggested answer written on the back of the card. Like Sharon's initial sentence, the suggested answer fit the criterion of being relational; it was "The woman is leaning *against* the tree." The therapist, however, interpreted what was being suggested on the back of the card as actively relational in a particular way. In the process of indirectly relating this to Sharon, the therapist set an exercise-specific standard for judging Sharon's response. We see that while there may be established or suggested standards for judging success, on the one hand, and a willing learner, on the other, the very process of relating the two itself destabilizes the standard. The process by which Sharon becomes an achiever is thus not simply a matter of displaying ability in relation to a test, or a matter of the clarity of a teacher's instructions; it is equally a matter of interpretations that arise from their ongoing interaction (Cicourel and Kitsuse, 1963; Cicourel, et al., 1974; Buckholdt and Gubrium, 1979a). Let us go on with the same therapy session.

[*Sharon looks at several picture cards and writes sentences for each.*]

Nancy: You know something, Sharon? You're doing really well because you're recognizing your mistakes. That's very important in learning. [*Pause*] Okay, now I'd like you to try these cards. They've got a bit more on them. Let's see how you do on these.

[*Nancy teaches Sharon how to write sentences describing the more complex pictures. Sharon struggles through several, finishing about ten minutes later.*]

Nancy: Ah-h-h. Whew! What a struggle! [*They both laugh.*] Good. You finally got'em. We've got a few minutes left before you have to go. Let's just do a few more and we'll call it a day, okay?

[*For a picture of houses on a mountaintop with trees below, Sharon writes: "The houses are above the treeline." The therapist is quite astounded.*]

Nancy: Wow! That was a really nice way of describing it. Ver-r-r-y good! I couldn't have said it better myself. Next time, you be the teacher. [*They both laugh.*]

[*Sharon looks at the next card, which depicts three men standing on a sidewalk with a house in the background. As Sharon thinks, the therapist puzzles over the card.*]

Nancy: Gee. I don't get that one [the picture card]. I wonder what they want you to say on this one? [*Turns over the card and reads the suggested sentence.*] Oh, I see what they want. Let's forget this one, Sharon. It's not really clear what they want from the picture.

Sharon: Should I do it?

Nancy: No. [*Pause*] Now let me give you some homework. I want you to do this page of words that you have to rearrange to mean something else. Okay?

Sharon: Okay.

Nancy: Let's do one first, okay, so you know what to do.

[*They unscramble the first word. Sharon says that she understands. The therapist comes to the second word that Sharon is to unscramble. It is: "Change* steal *to something that means* flavorless—_____.*"*]

Nancy: Sharon.... Uh, you can forget about the second one. Just skip over it and just do the others for homework. Okay? Just do all of these, beginning with the third one. When I looked these over this morning, I couldn't for the life of me figure it [the second word] out myself. I asked Bea [another speech therapist] if she could figure it out at lunch and she knew what the answer was. It was "stale." So I'll forgive you if you can't come up with the right answer on that one.

[*The therapist helps Sharon with her wheelchair. Sharon leaves.*]

In this excerpt from the proceedings of that day's speech therapy session, we find that, as before, the therapist is active in the specification of success standards. But something more is happening besides the articulation of standards in relation to the patient's performance. It is how the particular standard is being used in interpreting the correctness of responses. For example, is the standard being modified or changed by the therapist's own ability to successfully complete the exercises? After Sharon wrote "The houses are above the treeline," the therapist was impressed and openly complimented the patient. The therapist then commented that she herself could not have done a better job, which provided an *ad hoc* standard for evaluating how well the patient did. Later in the session, as the therapist explained how to do the assigned homework, she encountered a scrambled word that she could not unscramble herself. Because Nancy (the therapist again) could not unscramble it, she omitted the word from the series she had assigned to Sharon, which once more set an *ad hoc* standard for deciding which items should enter into the evaluation of the patient's performance on homework.

Beyond the practice of interpretation itself, we find that the specification of standards for evaluating patient achievement is linked with the evaluator's interpretation of his or her own ability to succeed in completing the exercises. A patient who otherwise might have successfully or unsuccessfully completed an exercise on the basis of the standards provided becomes an impressive achiever when that patient does better than the instructor could have done. A patient who otherwise might have attempted, successfully or not, to complete select exercises is not allowed to try them when the instructor judges that even the instructor could not have completed them successfully. The therapist's interpretations in this regard become integral parts of the patient's accomplishments: the therapist becomes a working standard against which performances are evaluated.

Consider how this happens in physical therapy. In contrast to speech, what is exercised and taught in PT are lower extremity functions. When a physical therapist evaluates the response or recent progress of a patient, several specifics are focused on: successful transfers, strengthening in select muscles, facility in walking, reductions in spasticity, and other signs of rehabilitative progress. While physical therapists describe progress in terms of what they take for granted to be normal functioning, as did the preceding speech therapist, they interpret progress toward normal functioning in relation to the concrete conditions of circumstances in which they describe such matters. "Normal" takes on its working meaning within the very process of meaning assigned. In evaluating the acceptability or normality of a patient's walking, the physical therapist evaluates normality as it fits this or that particular patient, not the idea of patient as such.

Like speech therapy, physical therapists specify standards by means of therapist-comparisons. Take a physical therapist, Pat, who meets her next patient, Ron, in the middle of the PT gym. Ron is a 20-year-old paraplegic who suffered a broken back in an industrial accident. He gets around in a wheelchair most of the time but has braces on his legs and is also somewhat mobile with a pair of crutches. Approaching Pat, Ron asks what they're going to do today, adding, "not the same old things." Pat jokes with him:

> Boy, oh boy. You guys....I don't know what I'm going to do with you. Are you guys always so bored? Am I a show or something? Maybe you'd like me to pull you up to the ceiling by the braces and ask you to do a couple of back flips. I think we'll do that. How about it? Huh?

Ron responds in kind:

> Look, you're the teacher. You all better get your behinds in check. Like I want to get out of here! I know all that jazz we've been doing for the last couple of days already. Let's get with it, *teach!*

Pat pauses for a moment, then suggests, "I've got one. Get yourself over to the table [mat] and we'll see what a really big guy you are."

Ron wheels himself to the table, which is a large platform about a foot off the floor and is covered with a gym mat. He transfers himself onto it and waits for Pat. She returns with a light wooden barbell and weights. She hands them to him and instructs, "Okay, Mr. Big Guy, let's see you do two sit-ups holding those. I'll bet you can't. I'm half as big as you are and I'll bet you I can do three." Ron snidely responds that "she's on." Pat climbs onto the table and holds down Ron's legs. Lying down, he positions himself and begins. Struggling to lift himself off the mat, he can't seem to make it.

> *Pat:* Come on. Come on, you big lug. I said you couldn't do it.
>
> *Ron:* Hey, gimme a break, will you?
>
> *Pat:* Look, I can do at least one of those and I'm just [imitating Ron] "a little lady."

[*Ron struggles for a while and, after a brief rest, manages to raise himself off the mat while holding the weights.*]

Ron (jokingly): There you go... little lady. How do you like them cookies? Pretty good for the first time, huh?

Pat (jokingly): Are you kidding! I did three of those on the first try... [sarcastically] "Mr. Big Guy." You're just huffing and a puffing like an old man. Maybe we should put you over on North Court [mainly for elderly stroke victims].

Ron: Hey, get off it, will you? You think you're really something, you know that. You can't even do one! I dare you.

[*Pat lies down next to him, taking the weights. She asks him to hold down her legs, and then does three sit-ups.*]

Ron: Okay, okay. It's my turn. So you've been practicing. This is the first time for me and....

Pat: No-o-o-o, sir. I did three the first time I did it.

[*Ron then picks up the weights as Pat helps him to the middle of the table. She holds down his legs as he tries again. He struggles, pauses, and manages to do four sit-ups with considerable effort.*]

Ron: So. What do you think of that? I'm going to get so good at this that we're going to have to put you in braces and I'll do the coaching,... little lady.

Pat: I'd say you passed. I'll give you a C and an A for effort.

Ron: Are you kidding? That was an A, and nothing but.

Pat: Don't get all hung up on it. You're going to work your butt off tomorrow. You were pretty good today, but compared to a "little lady," well....

[*They go on to other exercises.*]

As the session progresses, Ron and Pat talk over and describe Ron's achievement in each exercise in terms of two standards. One is an unspecified general standard, which they indirectly refer to in talking about what an acceptable performance should be. For example, when the therapist comments that some performance is not what she would call a sit-up, for example, she refers to some unspecified but established standard. In turn, the unspecified but general standard is clarified and confirmed when the patient responds in kind to the therapist's comment and reference. But the therapist also judges the patient's progress in terms of what she can or cannot accomplish in the situation. When the patient does better than what the therapist is capable of, the therapist is surprised, complimentary, or both (perhaps sarcastically so). When the patient does less, the therapist may be less enthusiastic. Such comparisons may or may not be linked with the patient's disability. In the last clinical excerpt, for example, differences in their sizes and strengths [big guy versus little lady] served as part of the joking background of patient/therapist comparisons. In other cases, the disability serves as such, when, for example, a comparison generates considerable surprise on the part of the therapist because, as the therapist remarks, "I've got full functioning in my arm and I can't do *that.*"

Wilshire people occasionally recognize the practical relation between standards and their specification, but they do so in a special way and do not dwell on the matter; with the press of organized clinical business, it is glossed over. Therapists' contribution to the specification of standards in relation to the working patient is treated, on the whole, as one of the hazards of clinical work, as the discretionary use for what is understood to be a normal part of the specific activity of working with individual patients. Being one part of such activity, the contribution is taken for granted to be something separate from the evaluation as such. For example, when the speech therapist compliments Sharon on how well she did in responding to certain cards, the therapist directs her compliments to Sharon's performance. The comparison with the therapist is not an evaluation of the therapist's performance, for it is understood, in the particular situation, that Sharon, not the therapist, is the one whose written communication skills are being evaluated. It is Sharon who is being praised, not the therapist who is being devalued.

Established standards are referred to by both patients and therapists. For example, when the patient asks what "the book," "the card," or simply "they" say, established standards are understood to exist. When a physical or an occupational therapist comments that a particular patient's range of motion in some extremity is "within normal limits (WNL)," she too references an established standard. Therapists and patients, in various ways, know that they take into account the unique features of each therapeutic session to make sense of general understandings. Indeed, they sometimes chuckle or joke about the very process of bridging the two, as happened when the speech therapist suggested that Sharon might well be the teacher next time. But the point is that it is taken for granted by both of them that, in the final analysis, Sharon is "really" the student/patient and the therapist is "really" the teacher/therapist. It is this working understanding—about their respective roles—that serves to maintain the separation between what each knows about established and *ad hoc* standards. Everyone knows, or comes to know, that both types of standard are features of practice, but they do not seriously recognize their interpretations as standards in their own right. What they understand about who each is respectively, more or less wittingly sustains the difference: it is only a joke that Sharon is the teacher.

There is another way to specify standards for judging progress. Therapists not only use themselves as a basis for interpreting specified or unspecified standards; they use patients too.

Patient comparisons are made in various ways. In judging a particular patient's performance on a certain day, a therapist may consider that patient's past performance. We ordinarily think of past performance as an obvious basis for judging someone's progress. Say that up to some point a patient was not able to peel a carrot successfully in the OT work skills lab and that one day the patient finally succeeds. We might think that she had made some progress in homemaking. But that judgment relies on the assumption that certain conditions for comparison are stable—for example, that the quality of the instruction and facilities was constant. While therapeutic sessions might have become more intense—the therapist may have given more detailed demonstrations of carrot peeling, for example—at the very least, it is taken for granted that later carrot peeling is being compared with earlier carrot peeling, not with earlier apple slicing or some other activity. But this is the point. While carrot peeling may be the subject of a therapist's comparisons of a patient's skill, it is assumed that carrot peeling as such is at stake in the sessions compared, but this might or might not have been so. This problem is glossed over in using the patient's past performance to interpret progress. On some other occasion, though, it may be directly recognized, such as when a therapist comments to another, "How do I know if she's made any progress? I don't even know if I was getting through to her before."

Consider this example. Until a particular homemaking skills session when a past patient comparison is made, what a patient and therapist had said to each other in the course of carrot-peeling instruction and carrot-peeling attempts centered on what the substantive meaning of each was. The patient continually asked the therapist what the therapist wanted done, while the therapist repeated the steps of carrot peeling with the use of adaptive devices like a pegged board to hold the carrot (for persons who have to function with one arm) and a dycem (nonskid) pad placed under the board to keep the board from sliding. The therapist repeatedly asked the patient what the patient was doing as the patient responded—did the patient understand what was going on? Did she know what was expected? Did she recognize the instructions? These "conversations" showed that it was not altogether clear to either therapist or patient what was being taught and learned. However, when the patient was finally considered successful, past performance was used as a comparison in noting that considerable progress had been made in homemaking skills. Whether the patient's past performances were carrot-peeling trials or trials of something else, the comparison takes the former for granted.

The therapist also makes use of the patient's future in evaluating performances. While the assumed standard for successful carrot peeling by persons with physical disabilities is the production of a peeled carrot with the aid of adaptive devices, when judgments are made, they are offered by particular therapists about specific patients. The standard is interpreted in relation to what are assumed as the future lifestyle prospects of the patient. The idea of what the future is develops out of the ongoing interaction of therapist and patient. The future cannot be specified by means of the patient's diagnosis. For example, while it is sometimes said that younger rehab patients, such as paraplegics, have brighter futures than elderly stroke patients, the meaning of "brighter," or whether one is considered to have any future at all, is interpreted in relation to concrete events.

The use of the future as a basis for judging a patient's progress arises on many occasions, such as the time when Karen, an occupational therapist, taught energy conservation and work simplification skills to Mary, a 27-year-old mother of two with spastic cerebral palsy and recent weakness in her lower extremities. On one occasion Karen and Mary were getting ingredients ready to make pizza in the homemaking area of the work skills lab. During this session Karen instructs Mary in the use of various adaptive devices to simplify the process. Because of Mary's difficulty in walking, Karen is particularly concerned that Mary learn how to save steps in the kitchen, something generally called "energy conservation." Karen shows Mary how to pile several utensils and items from the refrigerator onto a kitchen cart and wheel them, all at once, to the table where she will be dicing and slicing, thus saving the time and energy to fetch each item separately.

In the course of the lesson and demonstration Karen frequently refers to the need for such skills because, as Karen puts it, "You're going to have to do on your own when you get back home." Karen explains how each skill she teaches will be useful to her after discharge; she takes for granted that Mary has a future and will engage in activities such as cooking after she leaves the hospital. However, until now, the details of Mary's future lifestyle have not been specified; both have been engrossed in teaching and learning. As Karen explains how a kitchen might be reorganized to reflect the sequence of steps one would normally take in preparing food, Mary is enthusiastic: she remarks that what Karen has to say "really makes a whole lot of sense"—she had never thought about how simple cooking could be made—and that each of Karen's suggestions for food preparation was "really neat."

After Karen demonstrates various skills, Mary tries her hand at them. She is rather awkward at getting around, and while she succeeds in piling various items onto the cart, she has difficulty steering it about without running into the stove, the counter, and the chair that she left in the middle of the kitchen after she stood up. In the process of getting Mary to try out what Karen demonstrated, both Mary and Karen forgot to push Mary's chair back under the table out of the way. Several times, the integral activities of demonstrating work simplification (by Karen) and demonstrating how well one has learned (by Mary) intrude upon the very themes of conservation and simplification.

Mary finishes piling all the items she needs onto the cart and finally makes it to the table. Karen compliments her, "That was pretty good I would say . . . but I think we're going to have to work on it some more so you can do it more efficiently when you get home. If we don't, it's going to take you all afternoon just to get everything on the table." Mary is appreciative, "Yeah, I know what you mean. That sure does need more working on." But then Mary adds, "Oh well, I can get my husband to help me with it. He's really nice about it." Karen responds that she thought her husband worked. Mary then explains that he works nights and usually wakes up at about three o'clock in the afternoon. Karen is somewhat surprised by this, "Oh, then I guess we don't have to work on this all that hard. You're doing pretty well anyway." Mary then apologizes:

Oh, no! This stuff is really interesting. I really dig it. It matters to *me* because then I can help my husband get dinner. I was such a klutz before that I didn't think he wanted me to help out. He's always real nice about it though. I'd really like to help him. I'd really feel much better about it if I could. He really works so hard, you know . . . poor guy.

From this point on, Karen's and Mary's references to how well Mary is doing center on Mary's future self-esteem, not her independence in housekeeping. How well Mary does is linked to what they believe will best make her "feel good about being at home" when she leaves the hospital. Judgments of Mary's progress in OT are organized accordingly. In this case Mary eventually is considered to have made "great progress after just a few sessions," a consideration that glosses over the emerging and changing meaning of the standard against which Mary's achievements are evaluated.

Patient comparisons as standards for judging progress are not limited to the use of particular patients' past or future. Other patients also are used. When a physical therapist comments on a patient's ability to climb stairs with the use of a quad cane (a four-legged cane), the therapist may inform the patient that he or she is not making good progress, has not "learned a thing" that has been taught, or that some other patient, similarly afflicted, did much better. Or, on the contrary, a therapist may be highly complimentary, stating that another patient did not do as well under the same circumstances.

Patients do not passively accept any standard a therapist invokes. A physical therapist who exercises and taps (toughens) the stump of a left, below-the-knee amputee may exclaim to the patient, "Harry, I guess we're getting nowhere. You don't seem to have much strength there. You're not doing that well. Helen [another amputee] is doing leg lifts with weights and she's only been here a week." Harry answers, "Yeah, and she's a real horse too. She looks like she could lift an elephant. You can't compare her to me. Just take it easy. I got time. I figure I'm doing all right. I'll get there." Both therapist and patient argue a bit over the comparison. Harry succeeds in momentarily convincing the therapist that another patient would be a better comparison and that, when compared to that other patient, he's "not doing too bad."

Hospital folklore enters into the evaluation of patient progress in patient-comparisons. Many "remarkable" cases of progress and lack of progress in rehabilitation are known to Wilshire staff members. The young people who recovered easily from head traumas suffered in car and diving accidents are legendary such as a 16-year-old boy who entered Wilshire as a "near vegetable" and who was walking about the hospital in three months. There are legends among the more elderly cases as well, such as a middle-aged stroke victim, who spent a year in a nursing home as a "vegetable," and who, upon experiencing some return of function, was transferred to Wilshire and was wheeling herself around in six weeks, talking intelligibly with slurred speech. On the other hand, there are those unfortunate cases where rehabilitative promise existed but, because of complications, the promising patient died; for example, a "grand round" was once scheduled by the hospital's physiatrists, in which the case history of a 17-year-old brain-injured girl was to be presented to the hospital's clinical staff. There had been considerable optimism for some recovery, and indeed, therapists believed the girl stood a good chance of being "one of those remarkable cases" of progress in rehabilitation, despite her severe spasticity in all four extremities, with contracture of the left ankle and both elbows. Unfortunately shortly before the grand round, the girl went into cardiac arrest and died.

Remarkable cases and legends are known throughout the hospital by name. Long after they have been discharged, therapists refer to such patients. In talking about the progress of patients in one area of therapy or another, they remind each other, for instance, "...and you remember little Kimmy Cousens who came in like a wild animal and walked out of here in four months." And, Sybil Harrington, another patient, is spoken of with awe as that "remarkable little lady" who had broken her hip, was admitted to Wilshire hardly able to walk, and within two weeks, was seen dancing on the North Court with the leisure therapists. Knowledge of remarkable cases, particularly by name, is chiefly part of staff, not patient, folklore. This does not mean that patients hear nothing of such legends. Indeed, they do in connection with the patient-comparisons made by therapists. Only those few patients who have been in the hospital for lengthy stays (several months to a year) are likely to share the knowledge as folklore.

Remarkable recovery cases may periodically reaffirm their legendary status by visiting the hospital after discharge. On one occasion, in the midst of mid-morning therapies, a young man walked into the OT office. He was wearing a green workman's uniform. We took him to be a delivery man, until several of the OTs noticed him. They leaped to their feet and immediately greeted him by name, telling him that he looked "real good." They asked how he was doing and he responded at some length. As we came to realize in the course of the exchange, this young man was one of Wilshire's legendary remarkable recoveries. Later, one of the occupational therapists explained that he had had a terrible motorcycle accident with extensive head trauma. He had a near head-on collision with a bus, which she claimed he did not see coming because he was so drunk. He was transferred to Wilshire from a downstate acute-care hospital. At Wilshire, he experienced considerable return of function in all extremities in a remarkably short period of time. The therapists took advantage of this and pushed him into intensive exercise, speech, and avocational programs. He made rapid progress, was discharged, and soon returned to work. "And now," as the occupational therapist put it,

> Just look at him, will you! You'd never know he was ever all banged up. If you look at him, you'd think he was just another guy. He just walks right in here like nothing ever hit him. Kind of blows your mind, doesn't it? I've never seen anything like it. I wish I could say the same for some of those other guys in here...like Jim...I hope he makes it. You know what I mean?

In each department, therapists use legends as standards by which to evaluate particular working patients. Describing a patient's progress to the patient, a therapist exclaims:

> You've really come a long way in a very short time. I mean you've really learned a lot, Hattie, and I'm really proud of you. [*Turns to the observer*] Terrific patient, you know. [*Turns to patient*] I'd say you're going to be one of our star pupils. They're all talking about you, Hattie: "Hattie! The Legend of North Court." I can see it all now, all up in lights.

It is not unusual for therapists to describe a patient's progress or lack of progress by explicitly stating that the patient is "just another [named legend]." For example, one therapist may describe to another what the first believes are the dismal prospects for a patient and may embellish and concretize by comparing the patient with a dismal legend.

> I don't know if she [patient] is going anywhere. Nothing I do sinks in. It's hopeless if you ask me. I'm just spending all my time trying to think of something new to do...just so *I* don't get bored. She's just another Flora Oberg...like you stamped her right out of Flora.

Acknowledging the comparison, the second therapist responds sympathetically, stating recognition of what the other means and that one would not wish a Flora Oberg on anyone. The ensuing conversation makes it clear that it is the assignment to the working patient of the mutually recognized Flora Oberg legend which enables both therapists to know "precisely" what problems a particularly working patient poses, "precisely" what the evaluation of the working patient is, and why.

What does the practice of standard specification tell us about patient evaluations? Whether in professional or common usage, we know that conventional models of evaluation, in principle, take for granted that evaluation standards are not patient-specific or trial-specific. This assumption allows comparisons to be made among patients and between periods of individual patients' courses of treatment. Ideally it provides an unbiased rational for why, for example, one patient's stay in the hospital should be extended and why another patient should be discharged. Yet, while there are some well-established standards and, in general, the common belief that there are specifiable bases for comparison and evaluation, staff members still face the practical problem of linking explicit or implicit standards with concrete patients and their progress in rehabilitation. In specifying linkages, therapists interpret the meaning of standards in relation to individual cases. They make use of two bases of comparison in the process: particular patients and particular therapists. In doing this, descriptions of patient's progress are as much a product of therapists' activity as they are descriptions of what patients are or have become in rehabilitation.

Motivating the Patient

A perennial problem of all teaching/learning relationships is getting the student to have a positive attitude toward learning. Assuming the student can learn, that he has potential and is not retarded by some medical, psychological, or social barrier, teachers attempt to enhance learning by means of various devices. Some devices may be material; others are largely symbolic. As teachers, Wilshire therapists encounter the same problem with the working patient. Assuming the patient is medically stable and has some return of function, the therapist attempts to motivate him to learn what is taught. Whether the therapist's instructions are in walking, self-care, powerbuilding, talking, reading, the use of leisure, or in how to plan the future, successful learning depends on a patient who translates what is taught into personal functioning. How does the therapist enhance the patient's willingness to realize the skills taught?

One of the ways patients are motivated is by means of patient and therapist comparisons, as described in the previous section. While we spoke of such comparisons as practical processes by which therapists specify standards for evaluating progress in relation to the working patient, they also serve to encourage patients. A physical therapist who reports to the patient that the therapist could not have done any better at select exercises thus communicates that the patient's performance is appreciated. When the same therapist adds that the patient could even do much better than the therapist can do, the patient is encouraged to improve on the performance. A leisure therapist who coaxes a lethargic patient to "get it together" and use free time more constructively—like a much more handicapped roommate has done—communicates that the lethargic patient has more potential than others similarly handicapped but, because of lack of spunk, is going to "get no where fast." In the course of doing therapy, therapists continually make use of such comparisons to manage patients' motivation.

Another means of motivating the patient is the use of simple compliments, prompts, and threats in the course of therapy. Consider a therapist who is teaching a patient to do "wheelies." The therapist instructs the patient how to manipulate his wheelchair over various objects, and demonstrates how to negotiate a curb in crossing a street. Using an available wheelchair, the therapist sits at the edge of a wooden platform that is built six inches off the floor and turns her wheelchair about so that the large rear wheels are at the edge of the platform, which simulates a curb. Facing away from the floor, she shows and explains to the patient, who is seated watching her, how to descend to floor (street) level. The therapist leans forward in her wheelchair, firmly takes hold of two of the several pegs attached to the rim of the large wheels, and slowly pushes herself backward. During this, she explains that in leaning forward, her weight is more evenly distributed and will not cause her to descend the curb with as much force as if she were sitting up straight. She also notes that if she were to descend going forward, she would risk falling backward because the large wheels would fall to the ground.

Instructing and demonstrating, the therapist makes use of patient and therapist comparisons for encouragement; compliments also enter into the process. The therapist prompts the patient as well as offering both serious and lighthearted threats as ways of managing his performance. In this regard, take the following excerpt from a physical therapist's responses to a patient's first attempt to wheel down a "curb."

[*The patient (Don) has wheeled himself up the ramp of the platform that simulates a curb. He manipulates his chair to the edge, backward.*]

Janet: Okay, Don...now...okay you're doing fine. Now back up slowly.

[*Don lurches backward.*]

Janet: Whoa! Hold on there! Where do you think you're going? Not so fast.

[*She reaches out and stops him.*]

Don: What am I doing wrong?

Janet: You better watch what you're doing or you're going to back right into traffic. That'll be the end of you and your wheelchair. Let's try it again. Wheel back down and come up the ramp again.

[*Don repeats his approach to the edge of the platform.*]

Janet: That's better. Good. Go-o-o-d. That's real nice. Keep going. Keep going. Very nice. That's the way. [Don stops at the edge.] See, you can do it. I knew you could. There you go.

Don: Yeah...but you've got to be real slow. You could really get all racked up. Okay, now what?

Janet: Well, what did I show you?

Don: I'm supposed to lean over. Right?

Janet: Right...and back down slowly, re-e-e-al, slo-o-ow-like. You ready?

[*Don proceeds to back down slowly.*]

Janet: Come on. You don't have to go *that* slow or you'll never get down. The light'll turn red by the time you're down.

[*Don tries several times to back down but, each time, he nervously stops.*]

Janet: Come on, Don. Try it again...just like I showed you. You're not going to fall backward. We're almost done. I know you have it in you. You can do better than that. Let's see you go all the way this time. Try one more time and then we'll leave you alone. This is the last one, okay? If you don't try to really do it, we'll just have to do twice as many next time.

In this excerpt from a "wheelie" session in physical therapy, the therapist compliments the patient profusely when he does well. She tells him that he's doing "well," "good," and "very nicely." Such complimenting is heard frequently throughout a therapy session, indeed during and after every small portion of each demonstration of skill the patient is asked for. The therapist also prompts the patient to complete his performance. She prompts him to "come on," to "try it again," to "hold on there," and to "hold in there."

She also threatens the patient. In the foregoing excerpt, the therapist informs the patient that he better make some progress in
descending the curb or he'll have to exert twice the effort next time.
She threatens the patient with a promise of what his next session
will be like if he doesn't do as she suggests.

Compliments and promptings may be substantive, more than
the usual "good," "fine," "real nice," or "keep going." A compli-
ment may be tied to the poorer performance of another patient, or
may be linked with what is portrayed as the ideal patient. The
therapist invokes the ideal when saying, "Well, Suzanne, that's
about the best anyone could expect from a patient." or "What more
could a teacher want!" Other compliments are related to the
patient's background. A speech therapist practicing handwriting
with a former elementary school teacher who has suffered a stroke
compliments her successes with: "That's the kind of job only a
teacher could do. That's really good, Marian." Or, as mentioned
earlier in the chapter, a therapist might use a background commonly shared with a patient to add a personal touch to compliments. Promptings have the same range of interpersonal referential links. A patient is urged on because he or she is quite close to,
or not close enough to, some ideal performance. Prompting is aimed
at what someone of the patient's background, or of the patient's
and the therapist's background, would or could do.

While compliments and promptings are designed to motivate
the patient by encouragement, threats are designed to encourage
by setting conditions contingent on the patient's performance.
Therapists have various resources at their disposal which they use
in this regard. One is the control therapists have over therapeutic
programming. Therapists decide how much exercising a patient
will do in a particular therapy session, and they decide whether
to introduce new exercises. They also have some control over how
forceful their guidance will be in therapy, for example, whether or
not they will guide a patient's arm over a range of motion approaching pain. When a therapist exclaims, as one did in the last
excerpt, that what is to happen in the next therapy session depends
on how well the patient does in the present session, the patient is
informed that the therapist can make it better or worse, depending
on willingness to comply with directives. Of course, patients differ
in their willingness to be influenced by threats—some are rather
sensitive to them while others are not. Regardless of how effective
they are in shaping patients' performances, they are used by therapists as a means of motivation.

Patients respond to what they dislike in therapy, to what they believe are unwarranted excesses, in various ways. Some cry out or complain that the therapist is being too rough, too harsh, is going too fast, is unconcerned, among other things. What is most difficult for the therapist about such displays of disapproval is that they are so public (especially in physical and occupational therapy which are mainly conducted in two large, open rooms) and are patient-initiated. When someone cries out or yells, whether patient or therapist, it tends to crash through the routine clinical sounds and motions of the rooms. Should a patient yell, "Ow-w-w! Stop it, goddamn it! You're breaking my arm!", it can be heard by everyone present; patients and therapists are likely to turn to the fuss and look on briefly. It is not unusual for some patients to ask rhetorically, or mutter about, what is going on. The yelling singles out a patient and a therapist and, momentarily, puts them on public display. When the patient initiates a public accusation, it suggests that the therapist is doing something wrong. Should the therapist respond in kind, a public confirmation of the accusation is risked. Therapists, for the most part, attempt to contain patients' exasperation in as calm a fashion as possible, not attack them with their own complaints or, in some fashion, escalate the already too public scene.

The public feature of OT and PT is used by both therapists and patients as a means of control over therapeutic events. Not only do some patients attempt to manage what they disagree with in their therapists' actions by "going public," but therapists too may attempt to motivate or dissuade patients in the same way. For example, a therapist may attempt to encourage her patient by loudly complimenting him on his response to her instructions or demonstration. The therapist may call to the attention of several other therapists nearby the fine or uncommon progress that her patient is making. By the same token, the therapist may attempt to dissuade her patient by publicly noting what he should be doing, "like all the other patients here do!" Whoever initiates such public displays of control tends to initially define them and, thereby, use the public to serve his or her own ends. When such public displays spiral and "get out of hand"—which they rarely do—both patients' and therapists' efforts to thereby control therapeutic events race beyond their individual interests, becoming full-blown scenes.

Some patients respond to threats and other similar attempts to control therapeutic activity by refusing to participate in therapy. It is not uncommon for a patient to refuse to participate because, say, a therapist is, or threatens to be, harsh in exercise. A patient may claim to be too tired or ill and have his nurse inform OT, PT, speech, or leisure therapy, that he cannot attend that day or for several days. In time, refusals may lead the therapists involved to bribe the patient in another way. For example, a patient who refuses to attend his therapies because he's "too exhausted and must rest," may be told after several days, "you just can't lie around here like you're in a hotel. This is a hospital and, if you can't come to therapy, we'll have to discharge you."

Another resource at therapists' disposal is their indirect control over daily passes out of the hospital. While physicians order passes, therapists tend to request or recommend them (as therapeutically beneficial). On a pass, a patient may visit his family, be taken out to a restaurant or community event together with other patients by a leisure therapist, or spend part of the weekend out of the hospital, all without jeopardizing inpatient status. On the whole, patients like to get passes and therapists willingly seek them from physicians, who, in turn, rarely refuse them. Everyone can benefit from a pass. The patient has an enjoyable time and, for that, is grateful to whomever secured the pass, the therapist often reaping the patient's gratitude. And, because it is claimed to be therapeutic, the hospital does not suffer the concern of accounting agents over the patient's absence.

Because passes are valued by patients, they can be used to bribe them. For example, the hospital has an ongoing spinal cord support group that meets one afternoon per week during which paraplegic and quadriplegic patients learn about future prospects of daily living and employment opportunities after discharge. One of the two staff members who manages the group complains that there are always a few patients who refuse to, or who, after the initial sessions, don't show up for the meetings.

> There are always one or two. You know how it is. It gets to be around three o'clock and, all of a sudden, you can't find Jimmy [a 14-year-old paraplegic]. He hides somewhere, conveniently forgetting that he's supposed to be at his meeting. After one or two times pulling that stunt, we just have to put it to him straight—either he comes to the meeting or no more passes. He really likes to get out, you know. He's into baseball and now he makes sure he gets up here. It works. They just don't know what's good for them, but they soon learn.

Patient control by means of passes, of course, depends on the value patients place in them. There are some patients who have no one to visit outside the hospital and who have little or no interest in community events or activities. Such patients are difficult to bribe in this fashion.

Bribes are also used in more subtle ways. Patients soon come to learn, sometimes even informing each other, that a therapist's personal attentiveness depends on their willingness to cooperate, be hopeful, and make some progress. As one patient put it to another: "If you don't give a damn, she [the therapist] is not going to give a damn either. Hang loose and warm up to her." Personal attentiveness is not just a matter of benefiting from the individual interest of a therapist. It also refers to the presence of thoughtful or graceful conversation between therapist and patient in the course of exercising. It refers to the "other little things that make a difference," such as the breaks that therapist and patient take during scheduled therapy sessions in which they just sit around and engage in small talk for a while. It refers to the good-natured joking and sarcastic excesses that patient and therapist allow each other in describing their respective hospital activities. Personal attentiveness makes the difference between whether therapy is all business or equally enjoyable in a casual way. With patients who refuse to "put anything into it," therapists are more "all business" in their treatment and tend to "go through the motions." The same is true for patients who are considered cynical, who make sexual advances, who are verbally abusive, or who act in other ways that therapists believe interfere with their roles and their ability to make progress in the individual patient's rehabilitation. Such actions, in practice, are not merely factual features of patient's conduct; they are also filtered through what therapists themselves bring to therapeutic relationships. What cynicism is to one therapist does not guarantee a similar interpretation by another. What may be a sexual advance in one therapist's view may be the patient's way of getting attention in the view of another. Personal attentiveness is established or diminished by the ongoing relationship of each patient and therapist in doing therapy. Once spoiled, however, personal attentiveness is difficult to reestablish. There are some patients who never experience it.

In contrast to the need to motivate patients is the need to contain their enthusiasm. Therapists periodically come across patients whom they would describe as generally too eager to make progress. Eagerness also becomes a characteristic of some patient's motivation during select portions of their stay at the hospital. In excess, such patients are said to be "overresponsive."

"Overresponsiveness" describes a patient whose eagerness to learn, whose sensitivity to stimuli, is so high that he or she attempts to respond to what is being taught before there has been a chance to assimilate completely the therapist's instructions or at a more rapid pace than the therapist can manage. Such patients "come on too strong," as one OT put it, and tend to "take over if you're not careful." Like other descriptions of working patients, overresponsiveness is a patient condition that, in practice, arises out of the working relationship of therapist and patient. In attempting to understand the patient, the therapist has available the "language of overresponsiveness," as well as other ways by which to interpret behavior. What a patient is, in terms of motivation, is articulated through the practical application of such languages. While therapists use terms like "overresponsiveness" to portray the condition of a patient to various audiences, in practice, no reliable connection exists between the objective state of a patient's eagerness and a therapist's description of that patient's state.

Consider Laura, a 31-year-old, low-level quadriplegic. She has some functioning in both upper extremities but her forearms, hands, and legs are partially withered. She wears a urinary catheter, carries a urine bag under her clothing, and has been in a battery-operated wheelchair most of her adult life. At Wilshire she is learning how to transfer herself to and from her wheelchair, her bed, and other surfaces in order to manage a life on her own. Upon discharge, Laura expects to take up residence in an apartment modified for the independent living of physically handicapped persons.

One morning in the PT gym, Laura's therapist, Mitzi, presents Laura with a new plastic slideboard; it has tapered ends, is lightweight, very smooth, and has grooves that minimize surface friction and facilitate sliding. Mitzi shows Laura how to shove one end of the board between her buttock and the seat of her wheelchair, how to shift her weight, and how to slide down the board to the mat table. Laura watches and concludes jokingly, "Okay, buddy, I hope you know what you're saying. I'm not sure I can do it but I'll give it a try." Mitzi assures Laura, "Knowing what an overresponsive type you are, I'm sure you'll be telling me how to do it in about five minutes."

Laura very slowly manages to move her body to one side of her wheelchair, take up the slideboard, lean to her right, and place the board under her left hip. This takes about ten minutes. She is now settled squarely on the seat of her wheelchair with the slideboard sticking out horizontally from between the wheelchair and her bottom. Laura is out of breath and takes a break. She chats a bit with Mitzi, who has been coaching Laura while seated on the mat table next to Laura's wheelchair. At one point, Laura excitedly asks Mitzi a question about slideboards:

I just had a brilliant idea! Why don't they make these with some kind of seat that can move down these grooves? Right now I'm nearly dead and I haven't even started to scoot over out of this chair. It'd be easier... Boy, I'm not sure I have enough in me to get my tussy across there down this crazy thing.

Mitzi again assures Laura that she can make it and that, as far as she knows, there is no such thing as a slideboard with a moveable seat. Laura insists there must be and claims that she's seen something like it somewhere. She urges Mitzi to ask Nick, the medical supply salesman, about it when he comes in that afternoon. As Laura continues to insist and Mitzi claims otherwise, Mitzi finally gives in:

All right, already. I'll check into it if it'll make you happier. I know I'm right. You'll see. [*Shakes her head*] I don't know what we're ever going to do with you overresponsive types. You people are never satisfied. [*Chuckles*] Just slow down and let's try to do this transfer.

To this, Laura remarks, laughingly:

Get off it... "overresponsive" my foot... ha, ha, what foot? Where do you get that overresponsive stuff. You're just jealous because I thought of it before you did and I'm going to get the patent for it and make a killing.

They both laugh, banter for a while, and after a few minutes, Laura resumes her work to transfer herself.

Laura strains to shift her weight and push her body down the board, stopping now and then to regain her breath and composure. At one point she makes a valiant effort to make some progress when, suddenly, she realizes that she's pulled her urine bag and had a "spill." Laura is embarrassed and apologizes, saying that she's very disappointed in herself, and that she should have been more careful and gone more slowly, as Mitzi had suggested. Mitzi good-naturedly jokes about the incident and tries to overlook the accident, reassuring Laura:

Don't worry about it. Okay? [*Jokingly*] See what I meant about overresponsiveness.... Naw, just kidding. Look, we all have accidents. Just forget it. You're doing just fine. You're just letting yourself get away from yourself a bit, that's all. We all do that sometimes. It's okay, really.

Mitzi continues to assuage Laura in this way, normalizing Laura's eagerness. Laura, on the other hand, now insists that it's her over-responsiveness that's getting in the way of her doing a decent job of it. The half-hour session ends with Laura halfheartedly convinced of her overresponsiveness and Mitzi denying that there is a problem at all, claiming that she'll do just fine next time.

A different interchange occurs with Mitzi's next patient, Scott, an 18-year-old head trauma victim of a car accident. Scott has been a patient for five weeks and can now walk haltingly with the use of a cane. Mitzi and Scott enjoy a warm, friendly relationship but, according to Mitzi:

> Since he's started to get around here with his cane, he's into every-thing and not giving himself a chance to listen and to learn what he's supposed to be doing. "I want to walk, I want to walk," that's what he says. It's on his mind constantly, and he just trips over him-self or gets the cane tangled up in his legs. One of these days he's going to fall on his head and crack it open again. I tell him to slow down, but he doesn't listen. He's becoming so overresponsive.

That morning, Scott wheels into the gym, approaches Mitzi with a big smile on his face, and asks, "We're going to do some walking today, right?" Before she has a chance to say anything, Scott is up out of his chair and telling a patient seated a short distance from him to watch how well he can get around with his cane. At one point Scott informs Mitzi how *he's* learned a new way of using his cane, a different way to shift his weight around. Just as he is about to demonstrate the new technique, Mitzi tells him that she has decided they better practice in the "other room" today. Mitzi asks him to get back in his chair and wheels him to the room officially known as the "quiet room." It is a mid-sized room with a mat table and chair, located off the PT gym. It is used for overresponsive patients, patients who are easily distracted, or those who tend to get out of control during therapy. The room can enable a therapist to get a patient's full attention. Indeed, enroute, Mitzi tells Scott, "Look, you're too responsive this morning. We better get you some-where where we can get down to business, one on one."

As Scott practices walking (gait training) in the quiet room, Mitzi carries on a running commentary on his performance, point-ing out what is right or wrong about it. She makes suggestions and asks him to alter his posture, weightbearing, and movement. As in Laura's session, their conversation is filled with sarcastic remarks, banter, therapy talk, and talk about unrelated matters. About ten minutes into the session, Scott becomes rather defeatist about his performance, particularly after he nearly falls, as a result of getting the cane tangled between his legs. He repeats that he "can't do it," meaning walk normally. Mitzi reassures him that he can if he really tries. The session runs its course with therapist and patient dwelling on the issue of defeat and success. Walking behind Scott as she wheels him back to his room, Mitzi reassures him:

> Look, don't be so pessimistic. You're always looking on the dark side of it. It's not you. Don't think that. You're just going to have to face the fact that there's a lot to learn yet and that's that. I want you to pull yourself together and see you zooming tomorrow. Okay?

Mitzi leaves him at the South Court. On the way back to the gym, she comments:

> I don't know what I'm going to do with him. I wish I could get him to be more optimistic. He just never tries, never. I wish he *was* over-responsive.... But you should have seen him when he first came in here. He couldn't even get out of his wheelchair. Boy, has he made progress! He really learns fast. It's as if he can read your mind and he just does what you want—just like that. [*Sighs*] It's the weather, I guess. Kind of cloudy and gloomy. It makes them [patients] feel the same say.

If we seriously looked for instances of overresponsiveness in patients based solely on a formal definition of it, we would have difficulty recognizing it in the preceding episodes—and not because these are not clearcut cases of overresponsiveness or its absence. Rather, the difficulty in recognition would come as we confront the shifting meanings and use that the term comes to have in the course of topics, issues, and tasks taken up during and after each therapeutic session. As we have seen, overresponsiveness shifted in meaning from being complimentary at the beginning of Laura's session, to being something one scoffs at because the term is pedantic, and then to something that one uses jokingly in the service of lessening someone's embarrassment. Later, in Scott's session, overresponsiveness takes on other practical meanings. It is assigned to Scott's eager pride and is then presented as the reason for conducting the day's session in a more secluded place. Next it is used by the therapist to describe a desirable, rather than undesirable, state of motivation (for Scott, over-responsiveness would be desirable). Finally, and not uncommonly, a patient's responsiveness is linked to a situation totally beyond human control—the weather; the therapist provides this as an explanation for Scott's lethargy in therapy that day.

Chapter 4

Relating to Families

The image of rehabilitation that enters into staff members' relations with families is not as predominantly educational as it is with working patients. The particular image is linked with the various tasks at hand in relating to family members, some of which are chiefly informational while others are diagnostic, deliberative, even defensive. At times, for example, staff attempt to inform family members about various treatments and their general effects in rehabilitation, as staff do in the family support groups held at the hospital. At other times, staff are more specific in what they say to family members—in diagnosing a particular patient's problems, reporting the results of treatment, outlining individual prognosis, or providing professional advice about how to respond to the patient after discharge. The meaning of staff demeanor and language in speaking to families of the things and goings-on of rehabilitation cannot be understood apart from these tasks which, in turn, are worked through varied claims to being family or to being what sometimes are called "significant others."

"BEING FAMILY"

To some extent, the composition of Wilshire families reflects patients' age differences and conditions. Stroke patients tend to be elderly, in the range of 50 to 80 years old. To speak of stroke patients' families is often to refer to adult children with children of their own. On the other hand, the family may be limited to the patient's spouse. In still other cases, a few families are represented solely by siblings—the elderly brothers or sisters of a stroke patient who never married or is widowed and childless. Fewer still are those elders who virtually have no family. Among the latter it is not unusual for references to be made to living siblings whose current whereabouts are unknown. As an elderly, never-married man with left hemiparesis put it, "Yeah. I have a brother. The last time I heard—that was back around 1957—he was living in Chicago. He's got a couple of kids I think."

Spinal-cord injured patients and those with head traumas tend to be younger than stroke patients, a good number being under 35 years old. The families of those who are unmarried usually comprise parents and siblings while families of married patients are made up of the patient's spouse, children, parents, and siblings. The relevant family may also include extended family members, such as grandparents, aunts, uncles, and others. Because of the burdens presented by disability for some nuclear families, extended family members may become the patient's family for all practical purposes after the onset of injury or disability. The dependency status of the patient after his injury may shift the burden of his care and living away from strained parental relations to, say, more receptive grandparental ones.

Between typically younger and typically elderly patients is a mixture of physically disabled persons of various ages, from those with cerebral palsy to amputees. A typical family composition more readily comes to mind when one mentions a stroke or head trauma patient than when one refers to the family of a patient with cerebral palsy because of the more specific ages at which the former occur. Although these images do not necessarily correspond to the actual situation in all cases, they do nonetheless orient talk of, and about, the families of patients, the future problems which families are likely to face, and how families might have to be approached or dealt with.

While those who present themselves to staff members as respon-sible or concerned outsiders are often kinsmen, to limit "families" to kin would exclude those who, for all practical purposes, stand in for family, are spoken of in equivalent ways by both staff members and patients, and who come to be treated as, act like, and express the same concerns for the patient as kin might. The "family" of a patient might be a girlfriend or a boyfriend whom he or she may have intended to marry before the onset of a disability. The family may be simply a friend or a roommate to whom one has become personally attached. For example, the family of an elderly spinster may be another elderly spinster with whom the patient has shared a household for forty years. There are also concerned acquaintances of lesser duration who present themselves as the "only family" a patient has, such as the three or four elderly boarders who room in the same large house as a patient. As a social worker explained, "We interpret 'family' pretty loosely. It could be whoever is going to look after the patient. Sometimes it's the wife or the husband and sometimes it's just a friend...whoever, really."

The term "family" is applied by staff and patients to a variety of persons not necessarily related to the patient. Certain ones may be spoken of as "the real family," or the "only family" a patient has. Such references do not necessarily specify kinship and are just as likely to be applied to those who have no formal kinship ties to the patient. The phrases are often used to separate those related persons who, according to staff, "should" be responsible family members from the unrelated others who "actually are" responsible for the patient. To staff members, the latter are said to be the "real family" or the "only family" while the former are considered to be, say "just" the family or those who "should act more like a family." Patients likewise use the term. For example, a patient once introduced a young woman to us as his family. We took her to be wife or sister, but later learned that she was possibly a girlfriend, someone with whom the patient and several others of the same age shared a house cooperatively. The young woman regularly visited the patient, observed therapy sessions, brought her friends to visit, was the patient's responsible party to his social worker and therapists. The patient also told us later that his wife "could care less" about him and that she had "poisoned" his children against him. According to him, none of them was "what you'd call real family."

While staff members and patients use the term "family" in similar ways, they are not always in agreement about whom they specify as "real" and "unreal" family. A physical therapist, for example, may refer to a patient's wife as his real family and, in speaking to the patient, suggest that he be kinder to her when she visits him. He, in turn, denies his wife's status as real family because, as he puts it, "She's only after my money." As he explains, his real family is his beloved and concerned landlady "who's the kind of woman a guy goes out of his way for—like *she's* my family." Staff members in contact with concerned kinsmen whom they admire are likely to persist in speaking of them as the patient's family, despite the patient's contrary claims. On the other hand, staff shun the family claims of despised relatives and occasionally remind patients of staff's feelings about them. When staff's sentiments match the patient's, their conversations take the matter for granted rather than dwelling on it.

Outside acquaintances hold sentiments about, and make their own claims to, family status. A patient and his therapist may eventually differentiate between the patient's close kin and his real family while his kinsmen deny the differentiation. Thus two sets of persons may claim familial status and present themselves as such to staff members, which staff take into consideration in organizing responses.

Who the "real" family is to everyone concerned is not just a matter of semantics. It meaningfully organizes the ongoing practice of staff's and patients' relating to relatives and acquaintances. Definitions of "real family" or differentiations between "real" and "unreal" family are taken into account in interpreting a patient's relevant past and future. For example, the demands on the patient and staff of two alleged families may be used by staff members as an explanation for a number of related events and troubles, from the "cross-pressures" on the patient that "caused" his stroke to the difficulty of quickly compiling a discharge plan for the patient because it is unclear to whom he will be responsibly discharged. Such family complications make the business of relating to family members or outsiders far from routine.

To approach family simply in terms of kinship tends to overlook how the impact of the patient's disability affects claims to family status. The onset of a disability such as spinal cord injury means that the person afflicted no longer has the kind of bodily function that he and others once took for granted. A quadriplegic, for example, suddenly learns that he cannot depend on himself to cope with daily life in the same way he did before his injury. He now is mobile with the aid of a wheelchair. If his upper limbs are extensively paralyzed, he might have to depend on speech and oral functioning to signal and manipulate his environment. One quadriplegic young man in his thirties, Tom Martin, was outfitted with a battery-operated wheelchair that he controlled by sipping and puffing into a breath-controlled device located near his face. He was mobile in this way but depended on others for feeding and for the care of other bodily needs. What happens to family claims with the onset of such injuries?

Prior to a physical disability, to have family might have meant to have kin or intimate others whose relationship to the patient was based implicitly on his relative independence. The onset of disability brings the family face-to-face with the problem of dependence: Who, now, is the family to be in relation to a former able-bodied person? Before his industrial accident, Tom Martin's family was his girlfriend, a divorcée with children of her own. Their family life, of course, had been organized around their ongoing capabilities, not around the limitless incapacities that one might imagine either could experience. Their intimacy and caring took that for granted. With his injury, the horizon of caring and intimacy abruptly changed. How can Tom now express intimacy? Who is to care for him when he leaves the hospital? Can his "family"?

The questions arose frequently during Tom's hospitalization, both for himself and for staff members. Tom continued to refer to his girlfriend as his family throughout his stay, but staff members, particularly his social worker, were more doubtful. Referring to Tom's girlfriend, his social worker would ask, "Do we really think that now that he's a fairly high-level quad that she's going to think of him in the same way she did before? I'm not so sure we can depend on her to. Tom might have lost the only family he had, you know what I mean?" Staff never completely resolved the issue, which affected their relations with the girlfriend and with Tom. While Tom insisted that she still cared and would always do what she could for him, staff did not agree. Their idea of what she could do included more than what the girlfriend led them to believe she actually would do.

One result of this was the difficulty of speaking with Tom about his future. Tom was prepared to refer to his life after discharge *with* his family. While he was not specific about its particular arrangements, he nonetheless linked his future with the girlfriend. His talk about the future both grew from the understanding and confirmed it. When Tom talked of life after discharge, he spoke of his girlfriend: where he would be housed, where she would live, how easy or difficult the arrangement would make their continued association. In considering the possibilities in this way, Tom concretized and, to that extent, realized his understanding of the familial status of his girlfriend. Staff members, on the other hand, found it difficult to converse with Tom about the matter. As his occupational therapist noted, "You just don't know what to say to him when he talks like that. Should you just go along and agree with what he thinks? Or should you say what you really think? You've got to say something."

Another consideration regarding Tom's continued characterization of his girlfriend as "family" was how to present an actual future to Tom and others similarly injured. Wilshire Hospital conducts separate series of support groups for families and for patients with specific disabilities, and Tom participated regularly in the weekly meetings of the support group for cord-injured patients. The support group sessions are devoted to presentations by the hospital's various therapeutic services, each consisting of descriptions of the effect of spinal cord injury on particular physical or behavioral functioning; comments on the prospects for recovery; and advice about alternatives for community living. In the meetings staff members intend to present what they know professionally about spinal cord injury in their particular areas of expertise. For example, sessions are conducted on bowel and bladder functioning by a nurse clinical specialist in rehabilitation and one of the staff physiatrists. A session is devoted to the sexuality of the cord-injured patient, conducted by a husband and wife team of consulting psychologists. In each presentation, frequent references are made to the future. In one respect, the sessions are all aimed at offering descriptions of life to come for the cord injured. In discussing problems of finding adequate living arrangements and outside help, the family is frequently mentioned. What is difficult for staff members in the sessions is the problem of specifying for select patients, like Tom, what is concretely meant by "family" in the presentations and discussions.

In one session, on leisure living, a leisure therapist provided a lively portrait of what life with and without leisure could be for patients after they left the hospital. She repeatedly noted that, in contrast to their use of time before their injury, all they had now was time. While their occupation before their accident most likely was some kind of gainful work, their major preoccupation now was going to be the use of leisure time. She described what she called "constructive" and imaginative" uses of leisure time in relation to family and friends. When Tom spoke of his own possibilities in this regard, he too spoke of what he and his family might do together. The leisure therapist found it rather difficult to respond in kind. As she later reported, "I just didn't know what to say to the poor guy. I just said, 'Yeah, sure,' but inside I knew that she [the girlfriend] would probably take off when things got too rough." The therapist then explained that there was always a problem in presenting facts to some patients because "things are just not what people say they are but *they* think they are." As she summarized, "You either just have to talk to them straight and tell them what you think, or you go along and talk to them like everything's all right. Either way, it's not easy, but you've got to deal with it anyway and that's when you have to play it by ear. I'll tell you, those are the times when it's easy to just blow your whole image."

Staff found their relations with Tom's girlfriend to be awkward. Bringing her daughter along, she frequently visited Tom in the hospital. She spent time with Tom in his room, accompanied him to therapy, and frequently remained throughout a session. She wheeled him outdoors in the warm weather and sat on the grass next to his chair, talking and just passing time. Occasionally she spoke with the therapists about his progress. Asking the staff about him, she'd refer to him as *her* Tom: "How's my Tom doing?" "My Tom been good today?" After staff left her, however, they sometimes turned to each other and, out of hearing range, whispered disgustedly, as one OT did, "Did ya hear that? There she goes again. It's always 'her Tom this and my Tom that.' My Tom, my foot. She cares about him just about as much as I care about the dust in the corner over there." Another OT responded, "Boy, do I know what you mean. That's a real put-on. I wonder what her story about "her Tom" will be when he's ready to go home with her. Bet he won't be *her* Tom then."

The ongoing issue of being family—"familism"—is not just conversational. One not only talks about family or to family; talk organizes and makes activity meaningful and, in turn, is concretized by it. While staff members found it difficult, if not hypocritical, at times to speak with Tom and his girlfriend as if they were family, the difficulty extended to related events. For some time, Tom spoke of his eventual discharge to his girlfriend's household and care, something expected and confirmed by his girlfriend. While staff, again for some time, reluctantly confirmed this understanding in what they said to Tom and the girlfriend, they complained, as Tom's social worker did, "We just can't start to make realistic discharge plans expecting his girlfriend to handle him." Discharge decisions would eventually have to be reached and the social worker had a major responsibility in placement. Sooner or later, what staff members considered a temporarily expedient pretense would have to be faced for what it was, and spoken of as such.

Other matters are linked with the familism question. When a family support group for spinal-cord-injured patients is scheduled who should be invited to attend as family? In Tom's case, should it be his girlfriend or no family? If pretense is used in staff interaction with a patient to deal with a familism question, the pretense tends to break down in time as concrete realities and decisions press those involved to commit themselves to, and eventually make good on, what is said. For example, to explain to families in the PT session of a family support group that the Wilshire staff is readily available to assess—"more than willing," it is said—the household needs of patients who will leave the hospital for home or apartment, is to offer the service to all families, both alleged and real. Thus when Tom's girlfriend hears about this and asks for a home visit by Tom's rehab team, she asks his OT, PT, social worker, and possibly others to commit a morning or afternoon of work time to a family matter. In time, pretense becomes rather costly to those involved in its management, so much so that its escalation informs them that they soon must, as a PT warned, "...just face up to what we really think is going on and lay it on the line to both of them" (Glaser and Strauss, 1965).

Also concretely related to issues of familism are invitations to attend therapeutic exercises, family participation in all-hospital holiday activities, daily pass arrangements, outside responsibility in emergencies or in emergency discharges, and participation in family conferences. The familism question is far from merely definitional. Definitions soon run up against events and activities where resolution of the question is practical, an ongoing concrete but meaningful issue of relating to families.

Running through the issue of who the family is, whether in fact or fiction, are ideas about what the family should be. When staff members differentiate between a patient's actual kin and others, whom they characterize as the patient's "real" or "only" family, their comparison makes use of a standard. To compare the familial status of acquaintances, to describe the relative worthiness of those compared, and to specify the degree of familism displayed by particular persons, is to suggest a standard. Referring to a patient's children, a staff member makes a simple comparison when she comments, "I wouldn't call her son [the patient's son] family, but the daughter's all heart." A nurse describes relati ve familial worthiness when she remarks, "The oldest daughter has it over the youngest when it comes to being a proper family." And a speech therapist is rather precise when she claims, "Her husband is twice the family that any of the kids will ever be." Whatever the scale, staff members imply a standard in their comparisons and tacitly use the standard to evaluate social relations.

From staff's point of view, to be family does not necessarily mean that one has kinship ties with a patient. This is not to say that kinship is unimportant, for it does serve as a first rule-of-thumb for recognizing "real" family. In accordance with what the term "family" is commonly said to imply, when staff refer to family, kinship is taken for granted, until otherwise understood. In staff usage, to be related to a patient is, ideally and rightfully, to be family, especially closely related kinsmen.

There is a moral basis to familism. Notwithstanding kinship, in staff usage, to be family means that those to whom the term applies are truly *concerned* with the patient. When staff members turn to them, whether for support, information, teaching, or planning, they assume that family members will be genuinely interested in, and commit themselves to, the long-term rehabilitation of the patient. An unconcerned or unenthusiastic family makes it reasonable to ask, "Is this a family or isn't it?" or "What kind of family is this?" But to staff, concern also must be genuine. Staff distinguish between outside acquaintances, related or not, who "just go through the motions" and those who sincerely are concerned. While Tom Martin's girlfriend, for example, dutifully visited him and attended various family functions offered by the hospital, it was not enough to win genuine family status for her in staff members' eyes. Staff did not consider her to be genuinely concerned with Tom, just showing concern.

To staff members genuine concern is not only a matter of attentive responsibility. An outside acquaintance who regularly visits the hospital and takes responsibility for the patient's household and community affairs, but who does this coldly and without feeling is not acting quite like family. It is not unusual to hear therapists refer to kin as "just going through the motions." While such relatives do accomplish the functions thought to be a family's responsibility, their "hearts" are said not to be in it. Such a family might be perfectly capable of attending to the technical side of responsibility, but they are not seen as extending *themselves* to the patient.

Staff members see the expression of heartfelt care in two kinds of action. When someone weeps for the patient rather than for the envisioned burden he or she will present, that person is believed to be "feeling and caring." Not just any weeping will do, for it is not uncommon for staff to consider excessive and unceasing weeping as irresponsible and selfish. Only a measured expression of weeping signals caring. Although what "measured" means to staff members in practice cannot be calibrated in any objective, reliable fashion, staff's tacit sense of what is appropriate and fitting in the situation informs their response to those close to the patient as more or less family.

Certain phrases are also believed to signal genuine care. To describe what one has done to enable the patient to realize his personal well-being is to show concern. For example, when a daughter explains how she has "set up a nice room" for her stroke-afflicted father so that he can maintain his privacy when he returns to her home to live, she is perceived as being concerned for *his* personal needs. When a mother and father seek out information and advice from the staff in order to, as a father put it, "...build up his [a paraplegic son] image, you know, that he's still a man," staff hear this as an expression of selfless feeling for the son. Should information-seeking be part of a concern for the burden the son will impose on the parents, it might signal inauthentic concern. To staff members, being genuine family is being selflessly concerned.

Staff may become overtly pious when they feel plagued by artificial claims to caring. It is here that their piety makes use of parochial beliefs about familial propriety: unrelated men and women living together are believed to be cohabiting illicitly; having children out of wedlock is a sign of depravity; homosexual relations are a sin against nature; while recognized as legal, divorce is considered to be moral weakness. The moral hallmarks of family life are viewed and spoken of in traditional terms—work, hearth, and home. Thus, for example, in casting doubt on Tom's girlfriend's alleged genuine concern for him, a social worker snidely emphasized her disapproval by pointing out, "And what's more, he's just been living with her. That's not a marriage in my book. And she's even divorced...she couldn't handle it." In another instance, after conducting a home visit, a physical therapist reports doubts about whether a stroke victim's daughter is going to really care for him. The PT describes "...how the daughter acts and what she's always saying when she talks about her father when he's not around," adding, "and she's not really his daughter anyway. I found out that her mother's really the old girlfriend, you know, that old floozie that comes around to see him when she gets around to it."

Pious beliefs do not govern staff's relations with patients and their acquaintances. Rather, staff members make use of piety and parochial beliefs in discounting, or accounting for, meaningful evidence of familism. To know of staff members' pious beliefs is not necessarily to know which relatives and friends of a patient are, and which ones are not, considered by staff to be genuinely and rightfully family. The piety and related beliefs are explanatory devices, not objective diagnostic standards. In this regard, compare staff's interpretation of the family status of Richard Henderson's girlfriend with their view of Tom's girlfriend. Both men are quadriplegic and are in their thirties. Prior to their cord injuries, both shared apartments with their girlfriends, one together with his girlfriend's daughter. The girlfriends were alike in the regularity of their visits to the hospital and their participation in family-oriented activities. In explaining how Richard's girlfriend is "true family" (something Richard also claimed), a social worker made the following points in a review of Richard's progress to date:

> She [girlfriend] is really a genuine, caring person. You all know how she feels about him. There's not a selfish bone in that girl's body. He plans to live with her when he gets out. And I really believe they'll work things out. I don't think they're into marriage or any other straight stuff. They're pretty far out when it comes to stuff like that. But, so what? Right? [general agreement] What's wrong with that? It sure as hell beats a dumb, no-feeling marriage. And we've seen a lot of that. Right? She's real good to him—the only one he's got, really. You've got to give her credit. That's a pretty heavy scene she's taking on. I think they're going to make it, don't you?

The question of familism has no permanent answers. Anyone's claim to be, or not to be, family is subject to new evidence and reinterpretations. An outside acquaintance may suddenly be seen by one staff member as "family after all" but continue to be discounted as such by other therapeutic personnel. A patient may become more firmly convinced of select acquaintance's genuine care and concern as his therapists become more entrenched in a contrary position. New evidence brought to a therapeutic team's attention by a social worker may entirely recast the meaning of the team's knowledge of the facts in a case of authentic concern. In relating to patients' friends and relatives, staff members take into account what they currently "know" the latter's familial status to be and, accordingly, organize ongoing approaches and responses to them.

SUPPORT GROUPS

Wilshire staff encounter family members in two formal settings: support groups organized for the families of particular types of rehab patients; and family conferences in which a patient's therapeutic team, together with the family or significant others, review progress and discuss problems in the care of the individual patient. In this section, we consider image and practice in the support groups.

At present, there are two series of ongoing support groups for families, one for the families of stroke patients and one for the families of the spinal-cord injured. While the hospital services a wide range of physical disability, these two categories of disability maintain a constant and visible presence there. There are plans, however, to add support groups for the families of other disabled patients, as the need arises and staff interest develops.

The two support groups are alike in formal organization. Each consists of a series of six to eight meetings, covering particular rehab themes. Meetings are scheduled for one evening per week, usually for one hour. They are held in various areas of the hospital, depending on which service is presenting. For example, when an evening's theme centers on physical therapy, the meeting is held in the PT gym. Each meeting begins with a presentation by the evening's organizer and is followed by a question/discussion period. The themes of various sessions, along with session organizers, are listed in Table 1.

Well before the beginning of each series, a memorandum is issued to all departments and posted throughout the hospital announcing the dates of forthcoming sessions. Families are reminded, mainly by patients' social workers, that support groups are about to begin and that they are invited to attend. The family members of patients whose hospitalization is lengthy may attend repeated series. They become "old hands," knowing what will be said and the kinds of questions likely to be raised. Other family members attend sporadically.

The Meanings of Attendance

The regularity of attendance at the sessions may be used as an indicator of familism. When staff members discuss the problems they experience in working with families, they call on their knowledge of family participation to account for them. In discussing who the "real" family is of a stroke patient whose discharge planning is becoming urgent, staff members take attendance into consideration in deciding what to do. For example, in deciding whether to release the patient to his brother (which is the patient's wish) or to his sister (which is her wish), staff members consider, among other factors, the brother's and sister's support group attendance. A nurse begins a staff discussion by noting that the

Table 1. Themes of Family Support Groups

	Theme	Organizer
For Stroke Patients:	Pathophysiology	Nursing/Pastoral Care
	One Step at a Time	Physical Therapy
	Let Me Do It Myself	Occupational Therapy
	Listen to Me	Speech Therapy
	Seeing Half the Picture	Occupational Therapy
	Where Will I Go from Here?	Leisure/Social Services
For Patients with Spinal Cord Injuries:	Overview Spinal Cord Injury/Impact of Physical Disability	Nursing
	Adaptation	Occupational Therapy
	Body Image, Sexuality, Assertiveness	Psychology
	Personal Hygiene	Nursing
	Mobility	Physical Therapy
	Recreation	Leisure Services
	Health Maintenance	Nursing
	What the Family Can Do	Social Services

patient's sister attended the support groups religiously, nearly completing a second current series, while the patient's brother did not attend even one session. From this, conclusions are reached:

> ...and that tells me something. I mean when there's so much dif-ference between a brother and a sister in how much they show up... you know...at the groups and all. It's not like he [the brother] couldn't come. He's not working and he's got two good legs, just like the sister. That sure as heck is telling me something...like that brother doesn't, uh, care that much. To me, it does. I'd work on getting him

[the patient] to go and live with his sister. If you ask me, I think it's pretty darn clear that she's the one that wants him and, if you ask me, it'd be for his own good anyway.

The patient's occupational therapist responds and offers a different explanation. In contrast to the nurse, the OT sees the sister's regularity as a sign of being a nag and busybody, something which the therapist says the patient does not need. As the therapist points out,

So you can understand that a guy like Chester [the patient], who's lived by himself and managed by himself all his life . . . like he doesn't need her [the sister] attention. I've seen her around—we all have—and, yes, she's concerned all right, she shows up at all the meetings and all the rest of the stuff. But did you ever notice how nervous he [patient] gets when she's around? I'd put my money on the brother. We could think of the patient's rights, you know. I'd bet Chester wouldn't come to any of the meetings either if his brother had had the stroke instead of him. That's just the way the brothers are. It doesn't mean they don't care.

In working out a discharge plan, various staff members interpret and make use of family attendance, together with other information, in accordance with their varied understandings of attendees' motives and staff visions of the patient's future after discharge. Their decisions—in this case, deciding to whom the patient might best be discharged—are articulated out of the sense they make, alone and together, of what, among other things, attendance at the support groups means. In turn, whatever meaning is assigned by staff members to differential attendance serves as the factual, yet practical, grounds on which their decisions are said to be made.

A young wife who dutifully attends all the sessions of the cord injury support group might be said by a nurse to be "real family," "devoted," and "showing real concern and love." This might be supported by what the nurse feels she knows from her individual discussions with the patient's wife and contacts with other members of the family who visit the patient. The nurse offers both "theory" and "data" in support of her position. On the other hand, the patient's occupational therapist arrives at a different conclusion, also in theory and fact, seeing the wife's dutiful attendance as "really two-faced" and "just a good show" because, as the occupational therapist claims,

I see that woman everyday in OT. She's always sniffing around. She just carries on all the time about, "How am I going to manage him and how am I going to take care of this and that"...right there in front of him. You should hear it. It's sickening. If you ask me, I think she's only thinking of herself. She goes to the meetings just because she wants to see how she can get someone to help her with everything...to see if she can palm him off on DVS [Division of Vocational Services] or something.

There is no consistent relationship, in practice, between the regularity of attendance and staff's perceptions of familism among those close to the patient. The inconsistency, of course, also applies to the interpretation of poor or sporadic attendance. Parents who attend none of the spinal cord injury support group sessions are not necessarily considered uncaring. Yet attendance still serves to inform staff members of caring. Any number of accounts may function to cast nonparticipants as real family. It may be said that parents' long working hours make it difficult to attend every week. A social worker might explain that the mother keeps in daily touch by telephone. A nurse might mention that she knows the kind of parents they are because her own parents were "just like them." As the nurse remarks, "It's not that my parents didn't care about us. Actually, they were great and wonderful people, but they just didn't get involved in all that parent stuff, like at school and church." On the other hand, lack of attendance may be seen as further evidence for what staff members consider to be typical unconcerned relatives.

Attendance, like other actions, has no universal meaning in its own right. It takes on its meaning in its articulation with ongoing sets of opinion, ideas, and sentiments held by staff members about relatives and other outside acquaintances. To treat attendance or some other form of behavior as an indicator of the quality of caring, concern, or some other value would gloss over the practical meaning the behaviors are assigned as people take each other into account in their everyday affairs.

Who Attends

Occasionally, especially at the first one or two meetings, a few patients attend the family support groups with their relatives or significant others. It is not unusual, say, for parents to seek out their paraplegic son on the South Court for a visit before they attend their support group from 6 to 7 P.M. Parents or other family members may plan to have dinner with the patient in the hospital cafeteria and thereby make an evening of their attendance. Some make a point of having their evening meal at the hospital since they feel there is little time to eat their supper between the time they leave work and the time the support group sessions begin. Family members also seek out patients to find out where an evening's session is to be held and may be accompanied by the patient to the meeting place. These varied pre-meeting activities tend to make for initial patient participation in family support groups.

Wilshire staff conceive of the family support groups to be for the general benefit of family members and significant others. There are other support groups organized for the benefit of patients, such as the support groups for the cord injured. Staff members become somewhat concerned when, for one reason or another, patients attend the family support groups. To some extent it is a routine concern since this happens regularly at the beginning of each new series. Their concern deepens, however, when patients continue to attend, either at their own or their family's behest. As one father said, "I don't see why he [his son] can't be here. We have nothing to hide from him." While this may be true for select family members, it is not quite the case for staff nor for a good many families who are troubled by the "family matters" presented by physical disability and need to express their concerns and questions openly.

Staff's concern over the issue of who attends family support groups centers on the presentational problems posed when patients participate—practical problems of how to talk with, and respond to, two quite different audiences. (The presentational problems arise in somewhat different form with patient presence in family conferences.) First, the emphasis that dominates presentations to families gathered in support groups is a medical/interventionist one. The emphasis that runs through much of what is said to, and done with, the working patient is educational, as we described in the last chapter. In speaking with a cord-injured young man about his rehabilitation, a therapist is concerned with motivation, progress, and achievement. The therapist impresses on the patient that, while guidance or instruction will be provided, it is up to the patient to make progress. In speaking with the families and significant others gathered in a support group, the therapist may refer to similar matters but is not likely to present rehabilitation as chiefly a product of patient motivation and learning. Rather, the therapist informs families of what her service will do for the patient, how different interventions can, and ideally should, work to strengthen muscle, improve physical articulation, and enhance adaptability. Depending on the particular service the therapist describes, the source of improvement in rehabilitation is differently portrayed, but is nonetheless located in treatment.

Second, with the working patient, therapists do not dwell on what they sometimes call the "realities" of physical disability. For example, they do not remind stroke patients that, despite therapy, there is a good chance that their speech might be slurred for the rest of their lives. Rather, the speech therapist emphasizes the positive features, events, and progress in the rehabilitative learning process. A patient who asks about prospects for improvement is likely to be told, in one way or another, that it depends on how quickly he learns and on the strength of his motivation. While therapists do not deny the possibility of no improvement, they focus their talk with working patients around the good chances of, and factors that could make for, improvement. In relating to families in support groups, however, unrealistic hope is more likely to be entertained as a general concern, especially in discussions following therapists' presentations to the families of stroke patients. This does not mean that staff members are morbid or dwell on the matter. Far from it. Rather, on occasion, they make pointed reference to the "realities" of physical disability, the term being shorthand for a variety of concrete conditions—some well-recognized, such a paralysis, and others rather vague such as an old stroke—which may place limits on what can and cannot be done for the disabled patient.

Third, certain concerns thought to be family, rather than patient matters are discussed in the family support groups. Family matters concern the range of potential responsibilities undertaken in response to the patient's disability. Chief among these is whether to take personal responsibility for the patient's needs or care after discharge or to seek institutionalization. These matters are thus patient-sensitive, and staff prefer to discuss them, either generally or particularly, in the patient's absence.

Fourth is the question of patient decorum. While staff are prepared to deal with what they consider to be the inappropriate or uncontrolled behavior of patients in more private settings, like in the quiet room or in the family conference, they prefer not to have to deal with it in a public gathering. The support groups are settings where the hospital's care and services are presented, not its responses to individual problems tested. The relatively impersonal atmosphere of family support groups is changed by patient breakdowns, outbursts, and challenges.

Staff members express private and public concern over patient presence. Privately they complain to each other, before and during the support group proceedings, over what to do about this or that patient who either is brought to, or who attends, the sessions on his own. Before one evening's support group session began, the clinical specialist in rehab nursing asked a social worker, "Do you think Ralph's wife will wheel him into the meeting again?" The social worker sighed, "Well, I hope not. He was such a nuisance last time and it's so hard getting the point across to his wife." Ralph was in attendance at the first three sessions of the current series before it was made clear to him and his wife that the meetings were for family only. Ralph had annoyed the various presenters by, as one of them put it, "talking loudly all the time and not making any sense at all, crying out loud right in the middle of the presentation, and just annoying the hell out of a whole lot of people."

While many family members side with staff in their preference for a family-only series of meetings, this is by no means universal. A few family members want the patient with them or see no reason for excluding him. The variation among family members on this issue urges staff to take care to remind known violators of the family-only expectation, pointing out that many family members prefer this because they want to "talk openly and frankly" with other families and the staff about their concerns and problems without risking the embarrassment and hurt feelings that might develop should the patient be present. As a social worker explained to the children of a stroke patient:

> Look, I know you'd like your father to be there with you. But, really, I don't think it's a good idea. There'll be many things you'll want to ask about, things that are pretty difficult to ask when the person you're asking about is right there listening. I don't think you want to put your father in the position of wondering if you care for him now that he's disabled when you know that you just want to think out all the angles...you know what I mean? And, anyway, even if you don't think he [the patient] minds, what about the nurse and the physical therapist and the speech therapist and all the others? Do you think they can be as honest with you? They have to work with your dad everyday and it can be a real drag if he gets scared and gives up because of what he hears. It's for his own good, really. He'll be all right. You're more hurt by him not coming than he is. And it's only an hour a week anyway.

Staff attempt to prevent patient attendance in various ways. Their memoranda refer to the sessions as meetings for the *families* of patients. Family members are reminded of the place and time of a new series and informed simultaneously that the sessions are designed for family, not patient concerns. At the first meeting of each series, a staff member, usually one of the coordinators of the sessions, comments on who should and who should not attend, especially when patients are present. This is put as delicately and tactfully as possible. Nursing personnel on the P.M. shift are asked to dissuade the patients from attending; it is suggested, for example, that they be kept busy doing something else for that particular hour, especially those who desire to attend or usually are taken along by their families. The leisure therapists may be recruited to help toward this purpose too; they may, for example, be asked to make sure that organized recreational activities are held for the stroke patients where they reside on the nights the stroke family support group meets and that activities be similarly held where the cord-injured patients are housed on the nights when the latter's support group for families meets.

Displaying Hope

There are similarities and differences between the two support groups—for families of stroke patients and those of the spinal-cord injured—in how the future life of the patient and of the family's place in it are presented. One way in which the groups are similar regards repeated references to therapeutic intervention as instrumental in rehabilitation. Whether the point is made by speech, PT, OT, leisure service, nursing, social service, or psychology personnel, the respective services are described as professional activities that "can make a real difference" in the rehab patient's functioning. Therapeutic intervention makes the difference in whether the patient remains totally dependent or reaches maximal independence.

While certain physical aspects of the disabilities experienced by rehab patients are irreversible, this does not mean that no hope exists for functional improvement and a satisfying future, whether through adaptation, the strengthening of existing functions, or others' support. Hope lies in intervention. This contrasts with the locus of hope referred to in staff relations with the working patient, which tends to be placed in patient motivation and learning. Thus, as a nursing rehab specialist notes early in the support group series for families of stroke patients:

> Your mothers or fathers are here to improve and we're all here—the speech department, OT, PT—we're all here to try and make a dif-

ference in their lives. You're not giving up on them and we have great hopes for their living long and productive lives. We're here to really give them a workout. That's what a rehab hospital is all about. Like it says in this little brochure that you all received [reads from brochure], "People come to Wilshire Rehabilitation Hospital from throughout the state and the United States. They come to rebuild lives that have been shattered by spinal cord injuries, strokes, arthritis, amputations, and neuromuscular disorders." Like it says in big letters here, "The spirit of Wilshire Rehabilitation Hospital is upbeat, optimistic, promising a new life."

And, as a physiatrist explains at the first meeting of the SCI (spinal cord injury) family support group:

So you're all here to hear what we can do for your family member who has been cord injured. I'm sure that by now you all know the physical limitations, but there's no point dwelling on that. There's no point wrapping yourself up, or wrapping your injured relative up in a cocoon and just giving up. Let's make sure you all understand that the patient just doesn't convalesce here, that he's here for treatment in physical medicine and rehab. And, chances are, he'll improve. He'll get exercised and strengthened in OT and PT. He'll learn various adaptive skills...the whole ball of wax.

The hope that lies in therapeutic intervention is not just a matter of direct and indirect general talk. In both support groups, the therapeutic services display concretely the tools of hope in various ways: by naming, showing, and demonstrating. The sense of hope is concretized when, for example, a speech therapist refers to "melodic intonation therapy" as a device by which to develop the articulation of aphasic patients. An occupational therapist describes the potentials of work simplification techniques and energy conservation skills. She lists and briefly explains the function of the following apparatus: powerbuilders, deltoid aides, sanders, Herring tracks, polyform adaptive equipment, biofeedback. Together with many other devices, each serves to improve or enhance the patient's functioning. PT lists various lower extremity exercises and a few of the many special modalities available for treatment. The other special services, too, name and list their respective wares, from specific instruments for treatment to specific clinical processes.

On these occasions, names given to the various wares are more expressly technical and professional-sounding than in less public situations. The different ways of referring to the same objects or processes is at times openly bantered about by staff members. At such times it becomes quite clear that audiences are considered to be crucial in how things are described to portray the hopeful activities of physical rehab. In this regard consider the following excerpt from a conversation that unfolded as one of the authors casually discussed the use and operation of apparatus in the OT clinic with several OTs doing paperwork.

[*Pointing to a stack of fiberboard cones used for range-of-motion exercises, the observer asks the occupational therapist seated next to him what the cones are called.*]

Observer: Mary...See those cones over there on the table next to Don? What do you call those things?

Mary (OT): Well, let me see...What should I say? [sarcastically] Well, we could call them "R-O-M [range-of-motion] conical therapeutic devices." How's that sound? Fancy enough?

Karen (OT): [Laughing] Oh, come on. I think we can do better than that. How about the ladder [another range-of-motion exerciser]? Who'll try the ladder? Going once, going twice...

Sandy (OT): That's a...ah...a "calibrated, escalating, range-of-motion exerciser."

[*Laughter all around. All get into the mood of jargon one-upmanship. Several other devices are given professional names. Mary then temporarily breaks the mood.*]

Mary: [*To observer*] They're all for therapeutic activities of various kinds. Most of them don't have any particular names. We just use them. Whatever works. Like we've got the sander and the sanding table and, over there, the Coca-Cola beach ball and the vibrators and...get this...*theraplast! Ther-a-plast!* How do you like that one? All that is, is silly-putty, you know, like the kids play with. They [medical suppliers] sell it to us and call it "theraplast." And, over there, we work with the punching bag and the pulleys and the ladder...Did I say the sander? Yeah, I guess I did.

Sandy: Don't forget the DLM stuff.

Observer: DLM?

Karen: That's "developmental learning materials"...like the peg boards and form boards. And that over there. What's that called, Mary?

Mary: That's a deltoid aid. We use it on James. And over there is the Herring track. Sounds fishy, doesn't it?

[*Mock groans heard all around.*]

And Don [an OT pointed out by Mary] is doing an eval using the dynamometer and pinch gauge. You've seen those before.

Karen: [*To observer*] We throw a lot of that crap around when the families or the big deals are around... like Dr. Smart-ass. You should hear me when I give my thing in the support group. I'm on next week. You go to those. That's right.

Observer: I'll be there.

Sandy: You better put some of those fancy terms in your report or the readers'll think we're not very professional. You don't want them to get the wrong impression of us, do you?

Observer: [*Sarcastically*] I certainly don't.

[*All laugh.*]

On this particular occasion, when the mood is lighthearted and droll, words for things come to have a reality in their own right, separate from the things they are taken otherwise to represent. Temporarily, therapists speak of words (professional terms) as being the source of professional therapeutic activity. To use the right terms is to come off sounding like what one does effects what one claims. In their application, professional-sounding terms locate the concrete sources of rehabilitation in the objects to which they are assumed to refer, objects managed and applied by the clinical staff. The sense of rehabilitative reality produced by the terms-in-use, as Karen notes, is audience-specific: you use them in the presence of families and other important persons.

The names connected with objects and activities in rehabilitation are integral features—practical, connotative features—of interaction and circumstance. To sound professional is not merely to speak a clinical language. Realities are tied to what is assumed to be at stake in the organization. Sounding professional when the circumstance is lighthearted and spoofing, as it was in the OT office, lends an aura of absurdity to the rehabilitative hopes of apparatus and treatment. Sounding professional in a circumstance where the public orientation to rehabilitation is underpinned by assumptions of skill application and treatment offers a sense of concrete hope in apparatus and treatment.

The meaning of the therapeutic names or terms as used in family support groups stands in contrast with their intended meaning in the preceding OT office scene. In the support groups, words for apparatus and treatment techniques are not taken to have a reality in their own right; rather, they represent objects and activities that can be pointed to and demonstrated as rehabilitatively helpful. When an occupational therapist speaks to a family support group of stroke patients in the OT clinic, points to a piece of therapeutic equipment, and calls it a "ladder" or a "powerbuilder," she uses the name she gives as a communication device, not as a producer of rehabilitative images. She expects her audience to hear what she tells them in this way, taking for granted that it is not so much the words themselves that focus their attentions but the objects and activities that words represent.

Staff members take audiences into account in articulating images of rehabilitation. By various means, staff members publicly cast themselves and their audiences into different roles and organize their talk about rehabilitation accordingly. There are occasions, even within support group proceedings, that are similar in mood and understanding to the OT office spoofing. For example, in giving a presentation to family members gathered in a support group, a therapist may make a quick turnabout and, in an aside, poke fun at herself and colleagues for, as a physical therapist once said, "the big and fancy words we're always using for really ordinary things that many of you have around home and, really, could rig up and do yourself." In such asides talk and understandings resemble office spoofs. The humor and joking that run through "deprofessionalizing" asides inform their participants that while they are momentarily suspending belief in the medical image of treatment and wares, they are not being serious about it. The aside does not cast doubt on the image of rehabilitation but only on its expression—whether as part of the camaraderie of an office scene or to warm up to a family audience. Whatever its intended purpose, the lightheartedness supports this understanding in a way that a substantively similar but persistently serious aside would not.

The various therapeutic services extend their concrete displays of the hopeful prospects of treatment by showing and demonstrating apparatus and technique. In their presentations before family support groups, therapists not only name this and that, they describe the structure and operation of things and processes named. To say that a ladder in OT is a powerbuilder and to explain how the powerbuilder strengthens muscles and maximizes functioning is to inform one's audience that it is something the apparatus and its application do that effects rehabilitation, not what the patient himself does.

Each support group session normally begins with a formal presentation by a representative of a clinical department. Presentations are organized around two tasks that vary in relative emphasis from presenter to presenter: a listing of the rehabilitative priorities of particular service areas and a description of treatments. Some presenters spend the bulk of their time describing particular disabilities while others turn quickly to treatments.

Therapists describe disabilities and show their apparatus and treatment by means of slides and films, especially the presentations of OT, PT, nursing, and psychological services. For example, explaining to family members what various levels of spinal cord injury look like functionally, a physical therapist shows slides of low- and high-level cord injured patients in therapy. She shows a slide of a paraplegic patient doing bed transfers and one of a quad using a breath-regulated, battery-operated wheelchair for mobility (the "sip-and-puff" chair). The therapist may also explain the pathophysiology of cord injury by means of slides in which the spinal column is schematically divided into areas of injury and their consequent losses of function; sections of the spinal column are letter-coded and ascending parts of each section are numbered; levels of injury are denoted by means of the codes.

Therapists also demonstrate their wares and treatment techniques. Holding a session in the OT clinic, an occupational therapist has readily available for demonstration much of the apparatus and adaptive equipment used in therapy. In one OT session, a therapist, Bridget Kish, demonstrates "adaptive devices" used by stroke patients. She begins her session as most do, describing the relevant disabling effects of stroke: paralysis, visual cuts or hemianopsia (having only the left or right half of one's field of vision intact), apraxia (poor motor planning). Bridget concludes her introduction:

> So, as you can see, there are many, many ways that stroke can affect physical functioning. And for each problem, there are all kinds of variations, from one patient to another, which means that we really have to work on individualizing what we do for each. So, let's see the kinds of things that we do in OT to bring about more useful functioning in the affected areas. There are all kinds of things, things I can't even begin to list because we're always inventing new ways to treat problems.

Bridget then proceeds to draw her audience's attention to various parts of the room. She points to, names, picks up, and demonstrates the use of each item. At one point, Bridget refers to the problems that many stroke victims have in eating, one of the problem areas listed in the first part of her talk. Because stroke patients commonly have some degree of hemiplegia, their ability to manipulate eating utensils and to accomplish the eating function is drastically reduced. It is difficult for them to slice meat, which requires one hand to hold the meat steady while the other hand cuts. Such patients may also forget to chew or swallow the food that accumulates in the pocket of whichever cheek and side of the mouth has been affected by the stroke. Bridget picks up a rocker knife and shows how its curved edge can be used to cut meat with a rocking motion, requiring the use of only one hand. She also demonstrates how a plate guard can be used to keep food from sliding off a plate (the guard is a plastic shield that is attached to a plate, against which a patient pushes food with an eating utensil). Bridget demonstrates the use of other devices, among them: a dressing stick (a wooden stick with a hook used to pull clothing up and over one's legs and arms), soap on a rope (keeps one's soap readily available while in the bathtub), a bath bench (puts a person in a mobile position while bathing), a portable mirror (enables one to monitor the affected side of his face or mouth and avoid involuntary food storage or "squirreling" and the drooling caused by facial weakness).

Whether the presentations are made to stroke or SCI support groups for families, and whoever the clinical presenter is, to name, to show, or to demonstrate apparatus and treatment is to display the sources of hope for rehabilitation. Families can observe, with their very own eyes, the instruments and techniques of rehabilitation. To this extent, presentations are not merely rhetorical but factual.

The presentation of apparatus and treatment tends to be recipe-like. Presenters virtually tell families that, depending on the dysfunction, there is available a stock of clinical recipes to effect change in, or adaptation to, dysfunction. Turning from the problems of eating to modes of solution, Bridget summarizes:

> You can see how what we call "squirreling" can really be a constant problem for the patient and a source of embarrassment. For that, we place a mirror on the table near the patient's plate, in which he can see his face and keep track of the problem when it occurs.

In explaining to families how difficult it is for some stroke patients to pull on their trousers, another OT offers this recipe:

> They have a real hard time reaching down and pulling up. Well, we've got a real neat way of helping them with that. We show them how to use a pair of these pull-up straps. [*shows straps*] The patient clamps them onto his pants and then just pulls on them while he's sitting down, and up come the trousers.

Noting how spastic disabled patients become at times, making it difficult to flex and exercise their limbs, a physical therapist speaks of the "blessings" of hydrotherapy:

> It's not unusual for arms and legs to get all tight. You can really feel how hard and rigid their muscles become sometimes. Just feel them. If you put your hand on their arms or their legs, you can just feel how all tied up they are and they seem to be as hard as a rock. It can come from a combination of things. Sometimes we can loosen them up a bit by using the whirlpool; it can really be a blessing sometimes. They're lowered in there and it works to relax the affected muscles.

Recipes pervade the transition from problem presentations to treatments: "for that, we can do..."; "when that happens, we..." "someone who's affected in that way gets..." To describe them as recipe-like does not suggest that the treatments, in some way, do not effect rehabilitation. Rather, whether or not rehabilitation results, recipes cast a good measure of perfunctory certainty into what is presented to families as hopeful sources of rehabilitation.

From presenter to presenter, from topic to topic, each presentation serves to confirm a medical understanding of hope to family members. Key terms dot the presentations and reveal the image. Therapists speak of *treatment, therapy,* and *technique.* They refer to how they *assess* and, together with the physician, *prescribe* (order) a course of treatment. They speak of the prospects for success or *prognoses* in select cases of disability. They refer to their *clinical* judgment. They describe *progress* in treatment and cases of partial or full *recovery.* They highlight the hope that Wilshire, as a unique kind of *hospital* and treatment facility, can offer to those who otherwise might spend the rest of their lives in nursing homes or completely dependent on their families. Of course they caution against unwarranted optimism, but they still hold out a valid sense of hope for improvement through *professional intervention.*

Presentations are followed by a discussion period during which family members inquire about and discuss a variety of problem-related questions about their own disabled family members—how being disabled will work itself out in their individual cases and how they can respond to their member's disabilities. While addressing many general issues raised and developed in the presentations, family concerns tend to be framed in terms of particular experiences with disability. The way in which the particular is addressed and used in the discussion portion of support group sessions differs from its use in the presentation portion. The difference is linked with different images of rehabilitation and different senses of hope for improvement.

Presenting their wares and treatment procedures in the family support sessions, therapists frequently exemplify what they speak of and describe. Not only does a physical therapist, for example, describe gait training; she also shows a slide of Ethel Murray in gait training (a slide prepared by the hospital's audio-visual department). In exemplifying the applications of gait training to Ethel, the therapist refers to how the *therapist* does something or how *therapists* do various things in getting patients to manage their ambulation. The therapist's description centers on the application of the therapist's knowledge and skill to Ethel, who, in turn, learns to walk. Using Ethel to illustrate the principles and applications of gait training exhibits the medical image in one of its concrete forms. The therapist links Ethel's gait rehabilitation with the general principles and applications that had been described earlier. The recovery message is cast in terms of intervention: there is hope for Ethel (in particular) and it lies in rehabilitative treatment (in general).

When family members raise questions about particular hospitalized relatives concerning what the particular patient's prospects are for rehabilitation, or why that patient is or is not making the progress that should be made, staff members frame their considerations of the particular differently. They make greater use of an educational image. After a speech therapist describes the various clinical approaches taken to work with aphasia, the wife of a stroke patient asks:

> I was just thinking about my husband...I'm Cal Benson's wife. He's, uh, had a pretty bad stroke, as you know, and he's pretty aphasic, although I don't think his speech is quite as bad as it was a month ago. Well, what I wanted to know was if you think he'll ever get to be...you know, so you can understand what he's trying to say? The reason I ask is because I've, uh, watched some of the other stroke patients and some of them...like a couple I could mention... some of them don't seem to have made any progress at all really. I just wanted to know if it's going to be the same for Cal?

As other therapists do, the speech therapist does not respond to this in terms that question the principles of treatment and intervention but, rather, in terms of conditions that spoil their implementation, some of which are components of a teaching and learning image, such as a lack of motivation to learn. In response, the therapist first makes lighthearted use of what she calls "normal aphasia" to slightly dampen the wife's hope for rehabilitation while addressing the group as a whole:

> Before I, uh, begin, let me point something out. You notice how I said "uh" and how Mrs. Benson kept saying "uh, uh, uh" before... Yeah, now you notice... [*All laugh*] Well that's what I'd call a kind of "normal aphasia." We're all aphasic to some degree. You know, you've all had times when you... no matter how hard you tried... and trying makes it worse... no matter how hard you tried, you just couldn't form the words, or they came out all backwards. That's normal aphasia. Some of us are [*chuckles*] more normal than others in that way. To that extent, we can't do anything about it and we were never meant to anyway. It's just normal. It's kind of like we're not all as quick-witted, but that doesn't mean that it's abnormal or anything. I'm not hairsplitting either, although sometimes, there's a fine line... but anyway,... to get back to your question [*laughs*], there's the matter of who we're working with. If the patient was a, what you might call "high-level normal aphasic" before his stroke, you couldn't expect speech therapy to improve him beyond what was normal for him before. It's not us... believe me. Then there are some patients, like some of the ones that I'll bet Mrs. Benson has in mind, who refuse to learn. They're just not going to try and that's that. Well, on the other hand, what could you do if you were in my place? We can help, but if the patient refuses to respond, you can't expect much in the way of improvement. Sure, you might say, some of us [referring to the therapists] are better at it than others but ... that has a lot to do with personal preference... and you find that no matter where you go. In Cal's case... to get back to your question again... I expect gradual improvement. He really tries and I'm glad of that. Given that there's no further physical deterioration... and there's really no way of knowing that for sure, I think we'll see improvement in time. But we can't be too unrealistic about it. I don't think it's a good idea for any of us to think anyone can be perfectly normal again after experiencing stroke. Close to it, maybe, but not perfect.

The hope extended in answers to family members' questions about rehabilitation and progress in particular cases is often tied to extra-treatment factors: there is hope for return only toward whatever was normal speech for the particular patient under consideration; there is hope for rehabilitation only to the extent that the patient is motivated to make use of the information and training offered by therapists.

When principles of treatment and application are presented to families, hope is portrayed as lying in professional intervention (exemplified in particular cases). When families raise questions about similar matters in particular cases, hope is more likely to be linked to what the patient does or does not bring to the rehabilitation process. Indeed, in answering such questions, therapists may even explain that, in the final analysis, all hope lies in some return of function and the patient's willingness to learn—an understanding of recovery that is similar to the one that guides staff relations with the working patient.

The Limits of Hope

Displays of hope for improvement exist in all support groups, whether for the families of stroke patients or the cord injured. But there are also some important overall differences that center on contrasting understandings of the general limits of hope for select disabilities. Related to this are ideas about the future of the respective patients.

Age is a prime feature of patients' futures. Although when asked directly staff members respond that the hospital's aim is to strive for full and useful independence for all its patients, the specific meanings of "full" and "useful" are differentiated in the support groups and are repeatedly, but not formally, linked with age. In their separate family support groups, staff members make references to age, but it is not made the explicit basis of their vision of different futures. For example, presenters do not speak of being aged as a reason for ignoring issues of sexuality and disability. Rather, sexuality is largely omitted as a formal presentation topic and, moreover, is rarely discussed. This stands in contrast with the topics presented and issues considered in relating to the families of the cord injured. Age seemingly makes it reasonable to envision the future of stroke patients differently than the future of the cord injured. The difference justifies, but is also justified by, the topics and issues presented and discussed in the two support groups.

To describe staff's sense of the future for patients of various ages and disabilities is to construct and abstract the principles that organize differences in what is said to families about independence and responsibility in relation to their disabled relatives. Consider the sense of the future articulated through the topics and talk of independence and responsibility in the SCI support group for families. When therapists refer to family responsibility, emphasis is placed on the responsibility of maintaining the patient's independence. When a therapist demonstrates what is being done in the hospital to enable the patient to care for himself, it is suggested that families further support self-care as far as they are able after the patient is discharged. The responsibilities of the staff and the family are to train patients for, and maintain, independent self-care, respectively. The family is not as responsible for the continued direct care of the patient as for encouraging and supporting the patient's ability to care for himself, independent of family (parents, siblings).

The residential future of cord-injured patients, most of whom are young, is portrayed in terms of separate and independent households. Although a cord-injured patient may reside with responsible family members for a short time after discharge, the expectation is that the patient will soon move into separate living quarters, preferably an apartment, modified to serve special needs as required. An independent household is considered something a family should encourage, something that staff believe all young people rightfully desire. In one session, a physical therapist put it this way:

> I don't think you can expect to keep and care for your son or daughter at home. As you all know, all young people want to be on their own. For some, that means right now. For others, in time you can expect that they will want to set up their own apartments somewhere. It's natural and a normal thing and I don't think we should treat them differently because of their handicaps. Rather than feeling they're ungrateful for your assistance, you should encourage them to be independent. That's the aim of much of our work in the hospital. For example, we do home visits to check out apartments that patients want to move into after discharge and we advise them on how to get around and get along by themselves. Much of this is aimed [*smiles*], really, at helping them to get away from you—to keep them out of your hair...and to keep you out of their hair. No one wants Mommy and Daddy around all the time. And why should they?

Of course not all cord-injured patients are young adults. There are children and adolescents, most of whom are expected to return to their parents' households after discharge. Yet the ideal of independent living applies to them too, to be realized in the not-too-distant future. For example, in jokingly describing a 13-year-old paraplegic's erratic attendance at the support groups for SCI patients, a social worker referred to the youthful patient's eventual desire for independence:

> He's a real rascal. You should see how he works everyone of us around his little finger. He gets us to believe that he can't make

his group meetings...and, of course, we fall for it. He's got a real mind of his own and, pretty soon, he's going to want to be on his own. He's going to want his own apartment and, boy, is he going to have the girlfriends.

Families are advised how they can responsibly facilitate independent living. They are told to be ready and not to be surprised when it is mentioned by their disabled children. They are urged not to dissuade the natural urge to want to be on one's own, and are tactfully warned against encouraging excessive dependence. As a therapist explained, "Sometimes they [SCI patients] want to tie themselves to the old apron strings and just give up being on their own, but for their own good, don't let them do it. The thing to do is to nicely discourage it and build up their confidence." Families are apprised of various means of supporting an independent lifestyle. They are informed of the location of housing specifically designed for the handicapped. They are cautioned about what to look for in housing: the availability of large elevators, ramps for wheelchairs, barrier-free hallways and rooms, accessible appliances and household conveniences. They are told where to turn for help in support of their disabled member's independence, to the variety of public and private agencies available.

In the presentation, the OT embellishes a portrayal of future independence by describing the housekeeping skills required for living alone, without the constant availability of able-bodied assistance. Although any patient might be scheduled for therapy in the housekeeping and work skills lab—both young and old—the sense of purpose in scheduling younger persons differs from that of the elderly. It is more gainful and less diversional for the young. Describing how cord-injured patients are taught to make beds, do their laundry, cook, manage personal hygiene, and a variety of prevocational and avocational skills, the occupational therapist explains that these are the skills needed by all young people "in today's world." It is taken for granted that when the cord-injured patient is eventually discharged, he or she will take up the normal and active affairs of living independently and being usefully employed, not a sedentary existence financially underwritten and personally supported by others. As one OT noted, "The patient might not be able to do exactly the kind of work he did before, but we aim to get the patient to be the master of his own daily life." A former carpenter might no longer be able to build houses because his back was broken in a fall, but he can and, in staff's judgment, should strive to use his knowledge and the adaptive skills learned at Wilshire to organize gainful work for himself. He can do what many paraplegics with manual and mechanical skill have done in the past—he can develop a form of cottage industry and sell his wares at craft shows, consignment shops, trade fairs, and flea markets. Referring to work and the future, an OT reminds the families, "It can't be repeated enough, really, that these patients have a long and useful life ahead of them and they're going to want to support themselves and do it on their own. And it's important that you, as the family, understand how they feel about it."

In their presentations staff members portray the "active mastery" of the young cord-injured patient. Without knowing its formal academic connections (Gutmann, 1964, 1969; Krohn and Gutmann, 1971), staff members use a folk version of the "mastery style" approach to psychological functioning over the life course. A social worker speaks of the independent lifestyles that she has helped to build. She explains how the state Division of Vocational Services provided power tools for the home use of a patient who planned to make attractive and useful wood products—solid oak clothes hampers, carved wastebaskets, wine and spice racks. A long-time physical therapist recounts a case she heard about from a colleague who no longer works at the hospital. According to the therapist, a very intelligent and industrious young man, who planned to expand his father's hardware business into a local chain, injured his back in a skiing accident. He was paralyzed from the waist down and subsequently was admitted to Wilshire for physical and occupational therapy. As an in-patient, he became very interested in the kinds of equipment used in treatment. As the therapist told the story:

> You've all seen the stuff we use—you know, the weights and the transfer boards and the arm rests. Well, he'd be real, real interested in all of that...how this worked and how that worked and what we used everything for and where we got all the stuff. Actually, many of the things we make ourselves—the stuff you saw in the slides and in the gym—for our own particular therapeutic needs. Well, to make a long story short, that guy got out of here and started up his own medical supply business. He started up pretty small but today he's got a pretty successful company. He does all his business from his wheelchair and can he ever speak from experience!

Other success stories are sprinkled through the SCI family support groups. On occasion, the staff schedule a talk by individuals they call "real live, living" examples of success. A well-dressed paraplegic man describes how he made it in the business world, detailing the history of his climb. A female in a wheelchair explains how she managed to be a good mother and wife, raise four fine children, and help her husband everyday in the small supermarket they owned until he passed away. "Real live" testimony is corroborated with appeals to well-known legends, both local and national celebrities. Like the use of success folklore to motivate patients in treatment, staff members recount a stock of success stories for families to exemplify their vision of SCI futures.

The future envisioned is tacitly underpinned by a theory of personality. Some features of the theory apply to all young people; other features concern the particular traits of the disabled. Like all young persons, disabled young people see themselves as capable of limitless possibilities. They attack their worlds rather than let events develop on their own and adapt to them. After an initial but normal period of depression, cord-injured patients tend to confront their disabilities and, as a nurse put it, "try to do better than the able-bodied to show that they are just as good as the next guy." The sense of limitless possibilities among disabled young people is manifested in a desire to prove oneself, showing that one can be as capable as anyone, despite being handicapped.

Like all able-bodied younger people, the cord-injured are believed to be concerned with body image. It is important to them, for their feelings of self-worth, that they be physically attractive. Because they are visibly disabled, the normal problem of physical attraction is pervasive. Body image becomes a focal concern, especially in the case of adolescents and young adults, and staff relate the concern to the patients' developing sexuality—gender image and feelings of sexual adequacy. In support of SCI patients' concern, staff members inform families of the counseling available by psychologists, who specialize in problems of self-image and self-esteem in regard to intimacy and sexuality, to advise and counsel young patients.

In line with their theory of active mastery, staff attempt to develop the assertiveness of cord-injured patients—not aggressiveness, but assertiveness. Presenters show family members how an aggressive orientation to the world (a negative-active approach manifested by abrasiveness and verbal abuse) is less effective in negotiating daily situations than an assertive orientation (a positive-active approach manifested by tactfulness in speech and gesture). Staff also describe how a passive orientation is equally unproductive because, as a presenting psychologist pointed out, "When you always take this attitude, the world just passes you by like an old timer and that, my friends, as you know, gets a young person nowhere in today's world." A cord-injured person who manages to actively take hold of life and assertively deal with others has everything to look forward to, according to staff.

Now consider the future implicit in presentations to the families of stroke victims. The responsibility of the family contrasts with family responsibility for cord-injured patients. The family—real family—is portrayed as an available resource that, ideally, serves to maintain a maximally satisfactory lifestyle for their disabled member. Staff's message to families is that they must learn how to organize themselves collectively in support of the patients' care and provide him or her with a semblance of independence and privacy. Staff do not suggest that families abandon a goal of independent self-care for their disabled member. Indeed, family members are told throughout the sessions that they should get the patient to do whatever possible on his own as much as possible. However, as one therapist put it, "It's [independent self-care] not so much aimed at setting them up on their own, but more of an attempt to give them a sense that they're still their own person." Toward this end, the family's responsibility is, in the final analysis, to provide for, and continue to maintain, the stroke victim's individuality and feeling of self-worth.

The ideal future of the elderly stroke patient is one that is more concretely tied to family than the future of the cord injured. For cord-injured patients, the future is portrayed as one of independent living away from, and not directly responsible to, families. For stroke patients, independent living—in whatever form it develops—is seen as something critically dependent on continued family support. While the future may be one of maximal independence and self-care, it is not a future underwritten solely by the patient. The single or widowed elderly stroke victim, who maintained a separate and independent household before the accident, is encouraged to give it up for family-assisted or institutional living; the young, on the other hand, are encouraged to maintain independent living.

Staff presentations do not speak of the patient's future for very long before they mention the active and direct part the family should play in it; the stroke patient's future is understood to be the family's future as well. This contrasts with the future envisioned in presentations to the families of the cord-injured; here staff speak rather vividly of the patients being "on their own," ideally unassisted by their families.

Frequent references are made to the "burden" of stroke. The term is not unique to staff; it also is used by families and stroke patients themselves. Although younger patients also use the term, the meaning it has with respect to the elderly disabled differs from the meaning it takes on in relation to younger patients. The burden of stroke falls mainly on family members; everyone seems to "know" that. In contrast, the burden of cord injury is portrayed as a patient problem. All in all, the issue of being burdened is a more common topic of questions and discussion in the stroke groups. While spouses, children, relatives, and significant others of stroke victims frequently ask (sometimes apologetically) what the patient's symptoms will mean for the family after discharge, similar questions about cord injury are raised most typically in terms of their consequences for the patient's ability to manage his or her own life.

The burden of stroke places the family center-stage in presentations and related discussions during group meetings. There is a clear impression in the stroke group that what is being said is for the family's active use while in the SCI group, discussions are viewed as mainly for the family's information. In a nursing session, for example, families are presented with what the symptoms of stroke will mean for the bodily care of the patient. In various sessions, families are cautioned not to think of stroke patient's behavioral symptoms as mental illness but, rather, as normal responses to severe sensory deprivation. As a North Court nurse put it:

> It's very, very, very important that you all think of what's happening to the stroke patient as what might happen to anyone, any of you, if, all of a sudden, you had to go around wearing blinders or to hear things through an echo chamber, or whenever you had anything to say, it would get all scrambled up for you. Remember, it's not that he or she doesn't know what they want to say, that they're not the same inside. It's just that everything they want to say and hear gets out of whack. Of course that places a real burden on *you* as family. No one says its going to be easy for you but, at the same time, it's important to remember that we're dealing with stroke, not mental illness. For example, if a patient has a urinary accident, just remember that he didn't want it to happen and is quite embarrassed about it. It wouldn't be right to blame a person in this situation. And, of course, we're here to help you to get to know how to help your mother or your father or your husband along when this does occur.

When a physical therapist presents a session entitled "One Step at a Time," the families are informed that there is hope for rehabilitation and that it lies, to a significant degree, in what is done for the stroke patient in the hospital. But the therapist's display is restrained by references to stroke's limitations. As one therapist cautioned, "We can do many things for the patient—and so can you—but we have to go slowly and we can only go so far." Families are told that they should have a positive attitude toward progress but should not be unrealistic about it, that they should not expect the patient suddenly to be assertive and gain full independence; rather, the expectation should be to take "one step at a time."

In other sessions, from OT to speech, leisure service, and social service, a similar picture of hope is offered—a cautious optimism founded on familial support. OT shows families how they can be supportive in maintaining personal hygiene, how family members can caringly and resourcefully permit their disabled member to "do it himself." Like the nurse who cautions the families not to respond to the stroke patient as mentally ill, the speech therapist explains what is done in speech to enhance communication with those striken by aphasia and suggests how families might best "listen" and "hear" what the intentions are of their disabled member. Leisure and social services confront prospects for normal living. Describing their therapeutic and counseling efforts, they explain, once again, what family members can do in direct support of a positive future for the patient. Certain topics hardly are mentioned in the stroke support groups—gainful work, sexuality, assertiveness, and body image. These are assumed to be the concerns of the young.

The families of stroke patients are told to be sympathetic to the stroke victim because of unintended, sometimes inappropriate, behavior. Staff presenters often couple this with expressions of sympathy for the families themselves, who must cope with the difficulties.

> You have to put yourself in the patient's place. You have to feel sorry for someone who wants to talk but something goes whacko when he opens his mouth. I know it'll be hard sometimes—I really feel for you—but you just go easy and be understanding. It's a burden; it really is. Here at Wilshire, we don't give up hope and, if you really think about it, there's no reason for you to either. Your mother or father or husband or wife is still the same person basically.

For stroke patients, residence after discharge is usually a family household or a nursing home. Rarely is completely independent living embarked on. Staff members sympathize with families over the prospects of home care, and in describing the problems of nursing home placement, staff members sympathize as well with families over related burdens of guilt. In contrast, the sympathy extended in the SCI support groups shows concern for the difficulties the cord-injured patient will face in caring for himself.

The futures articulated in the two support groups for families are not the mere product of objective differences in disability between stroke and cord injured patients. Dysfunction for dysfunction, there are cord-injured patients whose disabilities are much more crippling that those of elderly stroke victims. On the other hand, some elderly stroke patients can hardly manage to accomplish the bare essentials of daily living. Both categories of physical disability are well represented by a wide range of dysfunction, from that commonly called a "vegetable" to near normal functioning. Cutting across variation in dysfunction is staff's sense of the futures of persons of different ages, normal or abnormal, able or disabled. For young people, the future is viewed as virtually limitless in its possibilities for material and personal growth. For the elderly, it has largely been spent—for some, spent well, for others, squandered.

The rare occurrences of hospitalized elderly cord injuries and young stroke victims support the significance of age and life-course understandings as principles organizing the hopes and limitations presented to families. Despite right hemiplegia and aphasia, a 33-year-old stroke patient is assigned greater hope for the future than an equally or less extensively disabled elder. Even though an elderly paraplegic woman is apparently more functionally able than a young quadriplegic, their age differences are taken into account in descriptions of their futures. The exceptions support the age rule: When a stroke patient is unusually young, the view of limited hope for strokes is not considered applicable; it still applies, however, to "common" strokes. When a cord-injured patient is old, the view of limitless hope again does not apply, for the same reason.

THE FAMILY CONFERENCE

The family as well as the patient's treatment team regularly participate in the family conference. At times the patient participates, depending on lucidity, the particular topic of the conference, how the family or staff feel about talking about the patient while present, among other presentational considerations. The patient's presence and the issue of familism both influence the image and practice of talk and demeanor in the conference. The family conference may be a fairly large meeting with several family members in attendance. For example, in addition to Rose (a stroke victim), her discharge conference was attended by the treatment team, her three adult children, and four young adult grandchildren. Her treatment team comprised her OT, PT, speech therapist, primary nurse, social worker, and a leisure therapist. Physicians rarely attend family conferences. Altogether, fourteen people were present. In contrast, the discharge conference of Kathryn (a stroke victim) was attended by her treatment team (excluding leisure therapy) and Kathryn's son, a total of six persons. It was thought best, by the team and the son, that she not be present, since one of their concerns was finalizing plans for discharging Kathryn to a nursing home, something they believed Kathryn might deeply resent (Gubrium, 1980b).

Conferences are scheduled for a variety of reasons. One social worker discussed their rationale in this way:

> Usually we hold the family conferences to help us get to know the family and work with the family on discharge. It's a good idea to have one if you're having a problem with a patient. It helps us a lot when we can get the family to work with us. The patient isn't always there...it kind of depends on what the problem is. Sometimes the patient's causing a lot of trouble and you just don't want him there when you're trying to figure out what to do about it. And some patients aren't very lucid and so it would be a hassle to have them sit in. I think the conferences are important because, you know, with these kinds of patients, you've got a future—not the same as before, sure—but you've got to prepare them for a different lifestyle and so you have to work with the family.

Another social worker commented further:

> All I get when a patient is admitted is this hospital admit form and maybe something like a single page factsheet on the patient from the referring facility. That's all...oh, maybe I've talked to the wife or one of the kids over the phone too, or something like that. Admissions sends the stuff over to me. It doesn't tell you much, boy. Then when I get together with them [patients], I find out about their family life, and a bit about what they did, and things like that. Usually I like to interview the patient alone because if you've got the family in here, they're all looking at each other and trying to decide what to say. I like to talk to the patient and the family alone. That way, you can get more honest feelings and you can check their stories out against each other.

The number of conferences that a family has varies considerably, depending on what information is available to report to families, how persistently the patient causes management problems for staff, families' desire for information about the patient, and the patient's length of stay, among other reasons. A social worker reflects on several of these reasons in describing how she schedules conferences:

> I don't like to schedule a family conference before the first staffing [a utilization review held within ten days of a patient's admission to the hospital] because there's a chance that one of the departments hasn't finished their "evals" yet. Sometimes you get pressured into it though. I schedule them ... when different services request a conference, like OT or PT or speech; there might be two or three family conferences. Once in a while there might be more, like when you're having problems with a patient or a patient's been here for a long time. We almost always schedule a conference before discharge ... to acquaint the family with future problems and all that.

While not required by law, it is considered desirable, even necessary, by some staff members, to have at least one family conference. Like pretreatment introductions and the ongoing talk that takes place during therapy, background information about the patient and the family gathered through family conferences is used by staff members to accomplish their work more meaningfully. They use the information both to manage their individual affairs with patients and to make more understandable what is said or reported to others about treatment and progress. A social worker pinpointed one recent source of troubles in this regard:

> Lately we seem to be getting a whole lot of patients with a lot shorter stays. I really don't like it. I mean you're just saying "hello" to someone, and you start to get to know the patient and the family and then you're saying "good-bye." It's really a problem because you just don't know what to think about how patients are doing and what you can say in your progress notes and in your assessments. You have to say something about why you think whatever happens happens. I think it's because we're getting so many CVAs [cerebral vascular accidents or strokes]. Most recent patients are old, and with a CVA, there's just not that much you can do. They're going to improve a bit up to a certain point anyway but that's it. There's not much you can do.

Preparation

Preparation for a family conference is not just a matter of working up descriptions of what is done for a particular patient in the different clinical services. The patient's treatment team is expected to report to the family about the effects of therapy, to provide reasons for progress or the lack of it, and to comment on prospects for the patient's future. Preparation for a conference consists of deciding how to assemble particular knowledge about a patient and describe it against a background of general therapeutic activity. While most team members are proficient at describing the latter in their respective areas—as they do in support groups—they cannot depend on general knowledge alone to sound competent in a family conference.

Should an initial family conference be scheduled well into a patient's period of hospitalization, team members have time to gather a variety of personal information about the patient and can complete the evaluations that serve as baselines for speaking concisely about progress. Notwithstanding issues of reliability and validity, having the evaluations available provides a basis for answering questions about change and progress. If team members have time to become personally acquainted with the patient, they can arrive at some kind of understanding about how he assesses the future and how motivated a patient is to respond to treatment; they can gather relevant life history facts; and they can gain insight into relations with family and significant others. Patient-specific information provides team members with a personal stock of knowledge to call upon in describing concretely the patient's rehabilitation to his family and in answering their particular questions.

Team members prefer that initial family conferences not be scheduled too soon after admission. Since any number of interested persons may request, even press for, a conference—from the family to the attending physician—team members occasionally find themselves saddled with a conference before they have hardly become acquainted with the patient. Soon after admission, a family may wish to know what the prospects are for rehabilitation. Some find it difficult, irritating, or unwarranted to have to wait a week or two before they are apprised of this. An attending physician who is badgered by a family may, as one social worker put it, "palm the family off on us to answer *his* questions because *he* doesn't want to be bothered. What the truth is, he doesn't know either and makes us do the dirty work of trying to sound like we know the answers when we don't."

Preparation for family conferences is a mixture of concerns with having something, anything, to say, and having accurate descriptions. For example, in the third week of a stroke patient's hospitalization, a speech therapist expresses concern to the patient's social worker that she, the speech therapist, "knows" that the family is going to want to hear more than "it's still too early to tell" or "the patient is making progress." The family is expected to ask questions about the amount of progress made in communicative functioning and how much is expected to be forthcoming. The speech therapist confesses that, because of her own difficulty in communicating with the patient, it has not been easy to evaluate him. She complains, "By now, everyone expects that you can come up with answers." The social worker sympathizes and suggests that the speech therapist estimate, to the best of her ability, how much the patient's reading comprehension and other communication skills have changed in the last two weeks. Taking the social worker's suggestion, the speech therapist presents the patient's two concerned daughters with an "exact" description of progress in comprehension, cautions them about the estimate, yet assures them with claims to professional judgment. The daughters hear the description as exact and respond accordingly.

Early in another patient's hospitalization, the team's occupational therapist claims to "know for a fact" what a stroke patient's precise level of functioning is in his upper extremities. Yet she also knows that she has just briefly met the patient and that there has not been sufficient time either to become personally acquainted with him nor to actually evaluate his functional capacity. Before a scheduled family conference the therapist claims, "I know exactly what those figures are going to be just by looking at him [the patient] but how can I tell his wife what they are when she knows— I told her—that I haven't even had time to do an evaluation yet? She'd think I was making them up." As the therapist suggests, being objective and precise is equally a matter of adequate presentation, of sounding objective and precise.

Everyone, in his or her own way, takes for granted that there are objective events and activities to report to family members, whether they are known or yet to be found out. It is also assumed that whatever is taken for granted becomes known by presentation. This makes the practice of preparation a matter of assembling a way of speaking about things. When a speech therapist notes that "I have to come up with something" for a conference, the therapist considers the knowledge garnered about the patient as well as how to present it to the family. Concern centers around possible repercussions of reporting to the family that, as yet, almost nothing definite is known about the patient's communicative skill: should the therapist come up with nothing and explain that it is too early to tell? Or provide precise, yet "estimated," measures and risk being heard as, and held responsible for, being definitive? And, can the matter of whatever may be considered to be objective information ever be completely separated from the meanings it will take on when presented to others?

Team members solve the substantive problem of having little or nothing to report to families in a number of ways. Before a premature family conference, an annoyed team member may rush to the patient's nursing unit to gather relevant information about the patient. The primary nurse is usually the first member of the treatment team to become acquainted and establish rapport with the patient. The nurse talks with the patient, exchanges background information, takes care of personal needs, has an initial estimation of functional ability, and usually interacts briefly with the family or significant others. Other team members therefore make use of the nurse's personal and interpersonal knowledge of the patient to assemble their own presentations to families in conference. For example, a speech therapist who has not yet met the patient may only be in receipt of a summary document stating that the patient is aphasic and that speech therapy has been ordered. The speech therapist knows the patient's name, diagnosis, and some other bits of biographical data, but does not know how aphasia is manifested in this patient's particular case nor what the patient is like personally. There is therefore no basis for reporting to the family what, in the therapist's professional judgment, will be the likely course of treatment or the prospects for rehabilitation. It is from the vantage point of a professional that the therapist expects to speak to the family; it is also from a professional perspective that the therapist believes the family expects, and deserves, comments on the patient. The speech therapist makes use of information garnered from the nurse to build a meaningful, personal framework around the patient's diagnosis—a framework that combines the therapist's general understandings of, and experience with, aphasia and its treatment with what the therapist learns from nursing about how it is, or might be, manifested in this particular patient. The therapist takes for granted that, in the forthcoming conference, the family will hear a considered, clinical report and not a hurried attempt to sound knowledgeable and competent.

When a team member lacks knowledge about the patient's family or the patient's experiences in other facilities, the social worker may well be able to "fill in" with useful information. What is known to staff about the patient shortly after admission tends to be divided between nursing and social work, nursing having a temporary monopoly on personal acquaintance with the patient and social work having familial and interagency knowledge, both of which may be cursory in their own rights. Should a physical therapist learn from the social worker that a family is "hopping mad" about the poor PT provided for the patient in a local acute care hospital, the physical therapist will take that opinion into consideration when organizing the information presented to the family about the prospects of PT at Wilshire.

Faced with a family conference in which they might otherwise have nothing to say, team members also make use of documents transferred to Wilshire from other facilities. "Workups" of various kinds accompany most patients to Wilshire—medical reports, psychological profiles, case histories, test results. When no one knows the patient at all, which is quite rare, information available in the documents serve as the substantive basis for an intelligent and competent report.

On occasion the problem of what to say is not a matter of a lack of interpersonal and personal information but of a particular team member being absent. Vacations, sickness, home visits, and other conferences, such as daily utilization reviews, keep a patient's assigned therapists from attending conferences. Other staff members substitute for the absent team therapist, usually someone from the absent therapist's area; less frequently, another team member substitutes. A substitute therapist makes this status clear to the family and typically bases the report on what was written on the patient's chart or in the assigned therapist's personal progress notes.

Team members may work urgently at gathering the semblance of a reasonable report when they know little or nothing therapeutically specific about the patient. They prepare, too, in similar fashion, perhaps with less urgency, when they are rather well acquainted with the patient. Regardless of the quantity or quality of staff's stock of patient-related information, signs of professional competence may be read from what team members report, such as the internal consistency of information presented and the language in which descriptions are offered.

Preparation is not only substantive; it also provides orientation information. In presenting their reports, team members take on particular demeanors that range over several dimensions: offensive-defensive, harsh-sympathetic, serious-glib, professional-lay, medical-educational. What team members come to know about the family through others or through their own experiences with family members informs the team of what they might better say and what presence they might best take on in the conference.

What is considered to be best is a practical judgment, arrived at both individually and collectively, and subject to redefinition in the course of conference proceedings. For example, what is considered the best overall attitude to take toward a repeatedly difficult family member quickly changes as team members encounter and interact with the member in conference. Or, in another instance, an informal decision to "lay it on thick" (speaking in professional/medical jargon) to a family because its members had been reported to be skeptical about physical medicine and rehabilitation, is forgotten when it is learned that represented in the family are a nurse and a speech therapist who, like themselves, articulate their "skepticism" in terms of the therapeutic difficulty of working with poorly motivated or pessimistic patients. As the meaning of family skepticism shifts away from challenges to professional credibility toward the challenges of professional rehabilitation, the team reorients the style and image in which it presents the patient to his family, from an initially esoteric and medical presentation to a plain and educational one. In this case, select family members are spoken to as the ostensible "co-workers" they are now known to be.

Familism is taken into account in preparing for the conferences. Team members consider what is known or suspected about the selfless care that significant others claim to have toward the disabled patient. Tom Martin and his girlfriend, discussed earlier in this chapter, were continual subjects of concern to team members in this regard. While the girlfriend expressed interest in "her" Tom's welfare, team members never ceased to believe she might be insincere. They knew of possible charges against her of prostitution. Several times, they were privy to Tom's own worries over whether he could still compete in his girlfriend's eyes with all the other men who were attracted to her. The staff occasionally commented that "different guys about her age" dropped her off at the hospital and waited for her while she visited with Tom inside. Team members were fond of Tom and they did not want to see him hurt and disappointed by the girlfriend. At the same time they were dubious over a community discharge, which the girlfriend explicitly offered to undertake in her own apartment. The team had made a home visit and, sure enough, the apartment building was wheelchair accessible and free of the usual barriers. In addition to the girlfriend's offer, of course, Tom was convinced that she was sincere and, in his own words, "the only family I've got."

Whenever a conference was scheduled for the girlfriend, team members wondered whether they could be open and sympathetic with her. With those whom they considered to be real family, they spoke frankly about both the promises and shortcomings of rehabilitation: they spoke of the teaching and learning problems of dealing with the working patient; they freely referred to the dependence of their intervention on the patient's motivation and ability to learn the functional skills taught and demonstrated; they explained how family members would encounter similar working problems and sympathized with them or the patient over the future difficulties that the burdens and/or tasks of maintaining independence would present. But they were also willing to outline the rewards of care, both in satisfying returns on achieving a modicum of independence and in patients' realizations of self-worth. Team members wanted to speak with someone in that way about Tom's future. Yet they rarely did during Tom's family conferences. They tended to be defensive when the girlfriend asked questions about Tom's progress, careful to describe their work with Tom as therapy and not teaching, rather elaborate in their use of professional jargon, and unwilling to put the same into layman's English. Indeed they sometimes would scoff at the girlfriend for not understanding professional terminology.

Conference events, of course, do not always unfold as they do in these examples. But they do unfold, and the assumptions, understandings, and descriptions around which they are formulated alter in quality as talk and circumstance change. And what are said to be, and heard as, the rehabilitative facts of particular patients' treatment are linked with on-going assessments of audience expectation, demeanor, and concern.

Presentation and Discussion

The format of the family conference is similar to the utilization reviews (see Chapter 5). There is a moderator who, in the family conference, is the social worker rather than the attending physician; the conference usually begins with a statement of purpose by the social worker. Participants may be told that the aim of a conference is to provide the family with the team's initial assessment of the patient and to offer an opportunity for family members to ask questions about therapy and the patient's treatment. Or the purpose may be to discuss with the family any difficulties that team members may be having in therapy, such as the patient's alleged sexual advances or verbal abuse toward staff, overresponsiveness, interference presented by family members in observing the patient in therapy, and the patient's reluctance to attend scheduled therapies. Each patient normally has a final conference in which discharge plans are discussed, where consideration is given to questions such as why the patient is being recommended for discharge, whether to finalize plans for a home or nursing home transferral, and how to finance arrangements for the patient's continued care.

The purpose of the conference established, team members present their status reports, in the same order they present progress notes in the utilization reviews. The image and practice of presentations are linked with ongoing assessments of familism, what is or is not known about the patient's disability status, and team members' feelings toward the patient being reviewed. The patient's presence also affects what is presented and discussed. As usual, the objective events and activities of rehabilitation as presented are articulated in relation to audience and situational considerations.

While staff resist having patients present in family support groups, they more readily accept a patient's participation in family conferences when they expect the patient will not unduly interfere with the proceedings. Staff do not as much present themselves and their professions in the family conferences as they professionally present the patient. Since conference presentations are made to the family, not to the patient, a silent or self-controlled patient typically is mostly ignored or patronized. While everyone is, more or less, aware of the patient's presence, ongoing conversation primarily is organized around team and family members. They speak about, for, and to the patient, speaking with him mainly when his feelings or thoughts are needed to embellish, certify, or fill in gaps in proceedings.

Two situations occur in which the patient is drawn into the proceedings as a full participant. One is the jovial or joking "aside" situation in which the patient jokes, or is joked with, about such awaited possibilities as, say, how surprising it will be to outsiders when they realize that the driver of a van who breezes around town is "really a cripple." Or the patient jokes about the rough and abusive treatment he receives daily in PT. As one patient laughed, "Yeah and, boy does she [PT] smack and bang me around. That's why I 'm black and blue all over, like that ad on TV that says, 'I'm black and blue all under' or something like that." The other situation is the aside in which the patient is the focus of sorrow and weeping. Hearing what is being discussed, an otherwise sober patient may break down and cry, in which case, those gathered in the conference turn to the patient with sympathy and caring concern. (Family members also weep in the conferences, both as part of patient asides and in the patient's absence.)

Many topics are discussed and questions raised in the conferences. Both team and family members continually "feel each other out," as a social worker put it, for what they have in mind concerning what should be done in, or expected from, rehabilitation for the particular patient under consideration. "Feeling each other out" is a continual conversational process in which team and family members search for, and infer, the varied images of rehabilitation to be current in each other's thinking and respond accordingly. What is said and meant in conference is not only a matter of what is known but, as a nurse pointed out, "It all depends on where they're [family members] coming from," referring to what the family is believed to understand about rehabilitation. The process is not fully explicit but is suggested by its participants' occasional references to what is meant by what is being said. This becomes a practical way of taking images into account while face to face with an audience.

Soon after the patient's admission, team and family members all will have run across a number of ways to think and speak about rehabilitation. They are exposed to its enthusiastic and concrete hopes, but they are also cautioned about its limitations. They hear and articulate descriptions in terms of treatment and progress, but also speak and hear of the crucial, indeed critical, place that the patient's motivation and learning ability have in progress. They all "know" that Wilshire is a hospital, that being made clear enough by the medical personnel and clinical environment, but they also "know" that what is most hospital-like about the place (the nursing units, nurses, attending physicians), in many ways serves as the background to other, more clinically active personnel and activities. They know that activities, rather different in application from nursing and doctoring, are the daily stuff of rehabilitation. In time, there is at least a vague awareness among most of them that much of what is done as rehabilitation is thought to depend on "return of function" or simply "return." It is never altogether clear to anyone, however, what the relationship of "return" is to staff's therapeutic efforts or to the patient's physical and psychological status. Team and family members' varied levels of awareness of these complex relationships among patient's and therapists' efforts, physical status, psychological outlook, and results lurk in their discussions and urge them to "feel each other out" in order to clarify the meaning of what is discussed and the question of how to present things.

Chapter 5

Third-Party Description

In 1972 Congress enacted legislation requiring all health care delivered under Medicare and Medicaid to be monitored by outside agencies. The mechanism chosen for this was the existing patient care review apparatus supervised by house physicians, which was now to work indirectly with newly formed local Professional Standards Review Organizations (PSRO). Being a third party, the PSRO was to bring quality control to Medicare and Medicaid and to contain rapidly rising costs. This was to be initiated in each health care facility through the regular review of cases, following local or regional statistical norms concerning appropriate admissions, acceptable diagnostic and treatment procedures, appropriate lengths of stay, and usual and customary fees. Previous legislation had required health care facilities to develop their own utilization review (UR) procedures. The establishment of PSROs did not replace existing internal review but added an additional layer of evaluation in the outside review of hospital UR decisions, case by case.

Wilshire's own process for monitoring hospitalization has several components, the primary ones being preadmission screening, the team or UR conference, and the review of extended stays. The central component is the team conference, where all staff members who work with a particular patient (the team) meet together to present written and oral reports on problems, goals, and progress in therapy and to make hospital stay decisions. The combined reports of the staff are then assembled into a document known as the "Team Conference Notes." These Notes are again reviewed in the hospital before they are subject to the scrutiny of the local PSRO.

In this chapter we consider the staff's descriptive practices as they work to prepare reports appropriate to and adequate for third parties. Third-party insurers, both private and public, use information in the reports in making payment decisions for services rendered as part of claims review. Data contained in the reports also serve accreditation purposes, another third-party function. What staff members report is assembled against background assumptions about the proper image and beliefs of audience expectations of treatment. While the events and activities described are presumably the same as those reported and spoken of to patients and their families, audience considerations combine in various ways to distinguish third-party reporting from other descriptions.

ADMISSION SCREENING

Mary W., a former nurse and current utilization review coordinator at Wilshire, is responsible for the day-to-day management of the utilization review. As part of preadmission screening, she reviews the chart of each patient seeking admission to the hospital, and then consults with a member of the medical staff. Mary maintains that she and the physician who review a case usually agree; initial differences in opinion or doubts are usually due to incomplete information on the patient. Mary sometimes consults with the heads of PT and OT when she has questions about the eligibility of a potential patient. They cooperate readily with her even though they are somewhat vexed at not having a formal say in admissions screening. If doubts are not resolved by consultation with staff, Mary may call someone at the patient's acute care hospital for more information. On occasion either she or a physician from Wilshire may even pay a visit to a potential patient. If Mary and the admitting physician either cannot decide or disagree on the merits of an application, information gathered from consultation and further investigation usually resolves the matter. There is rarely any direct or continuing confrontation.

Occasionally Mary goes along with a physician "against my better judgment." She becomes particularly annoyed with one and sometimes two physicians whom she suspects of admitting patients primarily on medical rather than functional criteria. While she does not confront a physician directly on his or her presumed interest in "purely medical cases," she does demand that potential patients be evaluated against a set of criteria for admission that Mary, as the UR officer, feels are rather clear. These criteria bar the following sorts of patients:

1. Those whose primary problems are not severe enough to warrant at least three hours of rehabilitation therapy per day.
2. Those who show evidence of physical, medical, or psychological problems that would interfere with functional progress.
3. Those who have completed an intensive, multidisciplinary rehabilitation program elsewhere but who have shown no significant change in physical functioning.
4. Specifically with regard to head injuries, those who are not responsive to verbal or visual stimuli, or for (hip) fractures, those whose onset of injury is over one month old, were not living independently prior to the fracture, who expect institutional discharge, and for whom discharge cannot be reasonably expected within three weeks.

Mary has found that charts and records transferred to Wilshire are sometimes "incomplete," "confusing," or even "misleading," and that she may need to check on their "facts." She described the difficulty in this way:

> I always look carefully at the records to see what the patient's problems are and whether or not they've made any progress at the acute care hospital. I also see whether or not they attend their therapies regularly, and if there are any clues to their motivation and alertness. But sometimes the records, how should I say it, don't tell all. Don't get me wrong now. I'm not saying that people lie, maybe "mislead" is a better term. The record says they can do this or that but when they come here they can't do any of it. That's why you need to get behind what the record says to know what's really going on. Sometimes the picture changes completely when you see the patient or talk to a therapist or nurse. They will usually tell it to you straight. They have their pressures too. For instance, sometimes a doctor is pressured by a family to word things in a certain way so that we will accept the patient or the nurses there might be anxious to get rid of him. There are a lot of ways to shade the truth and sometimes it's really hard to know what the patient's like from reading things.

There are occasions when particular Wilshire staff members help to construct the incoming records of potential patients, records which are later reviewed by other staff members for eligibility. A secretary in admissions, for example, told us how she sometimes tells callers from a referring institution what has to be in a chart or "how it should be worded" if the patient is to be admitted to Wilshire. The director of admissions also "assists" applicants. She sometimes advises callers what to say, based on her working knowledge of the diagnostic preferences of particular physicians at Wilshire, and she may highlight or downplay certain aspects of a case as she goes over the medical record with an admitting physician. On one occasion the director of admissions rushed out of her office to speak with a physician who was passing in the hallway.

Director: Oh, Dr. Jones, could you come here and look at this case for a moment. The woman's the mother of a doctor in town. She's in a hospital in St. Louis and he'd like her transferred here.

[*Dr. Jones glances over the chart.*]

Dr. Jones: There's not enough here for me to know what to say.

Director: I talked with the people in St. Louis and I think she's okay. She's been making some progress. I'll ask them for a complete file and tell them what to say if I have to.

Dr. Jones: Can we wait until it comes?

Director: I guess we could, but I've already told the son that I thought it would go through and he's planning to fly her here tonight.

Dr. Jones: All right, I'll okay it. Just make sure we don't get stuck on this one.

Director[*indulgently*]: Don't worry so much. It's bad for your health. I'll take care of it.

Mary recognizes that the problems she faces in evaluating medical records are not due simply to sloppy or inaccurate record-keeping. Those who prepare the records may have private reasons for "shading the truth." They may want a convenient way to discharge the patient, or the family may be pressuring someone for a transfer of the patient to Wilshire. Family members may be convinced that the patient can benefit from rehabilitation even though he or she has not shown much progress under existing care. Mary appreciates these sentiments and understands that a patient may indeed have more potential to benefit from rehabilitation than can be demonstrated in records of past performance. On the other hand, patients may also be far poorer candidates than their records show. This is why, ideally, she would like to see all potential patients herself before they are admitted. This is of course impossible, given the number who apply and the fact that many of them come from long distances.

Mary does postadmission screening of patients within 24 hours of their arrival. This is a formal part of the utilization review process. The postadmission review affords Mary the opportunity to find out what the preadmission records mean and to identify those who should not have been admitted in the first place. While she may alert the staff to a problem, mistakes are not easy to correct. It is difficult to tell the patient and the family that the client cannot tolerate an intensive therapy program after the patient has been duly admitted. The hospital also risks denial of payment if an inappropriate admission is acknowledged. Mary describes how she handles a situation of this sort.

> We are trying to make more use of trial admissions. That way, if things don't work out, we don't have such a problem with the family or the insurance company. But when we do make a mistake and admit a patient who isn't a good candidate for rehabilitation, we keep them, at least for a while. Even if we feel they won't make much progress toward real independence, we can always find some short-range goals to justify their stay for a while. Then we jump on the social worker to get moving with discharge planning. We don't want to keep them any longer than we have to.

Other, unpredictable, factors can serve to "correct" incoming medical records. Some patients experience unexpected return of function, almost overnight, while others regress for unknown reasons. Motivation can wax and wane. Transfer to Wilshire is a rebirth to some but may be a sign of failure to others. A change in family situation, a new roommate, or a different doctor or nurse can also make a difference. Staff recount stories of patients whom they originally thought should not have been admitted but who eventually made good progress and patients who made little headway despite their potential. These so-called "unknowns" inform Mary and other staff members of the continuing interpretive perils involved in making sense of records—perils that sometimes do, and sometimes do not, justify taking chances on admission.

The staff at Wilshire are confident that they can tighten and systematize the admission process, hoping to make their criteria clearer and more objective. The recently expanded guidelines for the admission of hip fracture patients are cited as an example of what they hope to accomplish. With clearer guidelines, staff expect to do a better job of screening potential patients, and referring hospitals and physicians will have a better idea of the kinds of patients that are eligible for treatment at Wilshire.

While Mary and her colleagues favor more exact specification of admission criteria, they do not believe that the procedure could ever be so exact that a computer could take over the admission-reviewing function. This would be a mistake, they believe, because they recognize the value of what is variously described as "professional discretion," "experience," "insight," and "intuition"— all skills that help them read and understand more than is immediately available in patients' records.

THE UTILIZATION REVIEW FORMAT

Before turning to the practice of the team's utilization review, let us describe its format. The format has three parts: the completion of Clinical Progress Notes; the team conference proper, where the progress reported in Notes and in individual staff members' testimony is discussed; and reviews of recommendations for extended stay.

Progress Notes and Team Conferences

Progress Notes are discussed by the patients' therapy team in the team conference. A conference is scheduled for each patient not later than ten days after admission and every two weeks thereafter. Each conference is chaired by a physician. Only his or her patients are considered, unless a physician is substituting for a colleague on vacation. Anywhere from three to sixteen patients are scheduled for a particular day's conference, depending on the physician's caseload. Also in attendance are a physical and occupational therapist, a nurse, a social worker, sometimes a speech therapist, and occasionally a consulting psychologist.

Each team member is expected to prepare a written "Clinical Progress Note" in advance of the conference, for which a half-page form in triplicate is provided. Narrow spaces at the top and bottom are for recording such information as the patient's and physician's names, as well as a code for rating level of care for PT, OT, and nursing—ranging through eight levels, from "totally dependent" to "independent". There is also a four-level code for rating the severity of the patient's problems in the areas of speech, social services, leisure services, and nursing. The main body of the Note is reserved for a written description of progress prepared by the therapist. The narrative sometimes spills over onto two or even three additional forms. The attending physician does not prepare a note for the conference but, rather, writes or dictates a brief concluding summary that is added later by a medical records secretary to the two- or three-page "Team Conference Notes" which she prepares, containing all the individually written Progress Notes. (All Team Conference Notes and selected chart records are submitted for claims reviews to third-party payers *after* all services have been provided and the patient has been discharged from the hospital.)

The nursing staff reports first. A nurse reads a prepared Note that centers on the patient's medical status. Among other things, she describes the patient's current medication, blood sugar levels, swelling, sores, and bowel and bladder management. She may also comment on the patient's sleeping and eating habits and personal hygiene. The nurse may report on the patient's dependency status, including how much and what kind of assistance he requires for dressing, feeding, and mobility, and whether supervision and behavioral cues are necessary. Notes are frequently interspersed with references to the patient's "reality orientation," motivation, and recent changes in any of the above concerns. Finally, the nurse lists projected goals for the patient, such as improving bowel and bladder functioning, teaching personal safety and hygiene skills, and building confidence and motivation.

Normally PT and then OT report next. PTs and OTs commonly organize their notes according to the so-called SOAP format. Widely used in health care facilities, the acronym stands for symptoms or subjective data (S), objective findings (O), assessment (A), and plan (P). As noted in a SOAP guideline circulated to staff members, the contents should be as follows:

S—Documentation of the chief complaint concerning the problem.
O—Quantitative statements that can be measured or graded and can be reproduced.
A—Documentation of the patient's potential based on objective findings and professional judgment; long- and short-range goals to be achieved.
P—Specific statement of how the problem is to be solved. This might include further testing procedures, an outline of the therapeutic program and/or educational sessions for the patient or his family.

While the therapists often struggle with the interpretation of the guideline, their finished Progress Notes and reports provide little or no evidence of it. The Subjective section includes information on such things as the patient's motivation, orientation, fears, and complaints. Sometimes family members are discussed. The Objective section that follows sometimes has details obtained from the initial evaluation concerning strength, range of motion, balance, ability to do "transfers," or related matters. In other instances reference may be made to the fact that the evaluations are available in the patient's chart and only a summary of major problems is provided, along with brief assessments of recent gains or losses and conditions that complicate the situation such as spasticity or poor safety techniques. The next section, Assessment, is used for a variety of purposes. If the patient is newly admitted, the therapist may discuss his suitability for teaching, how much progress is likely, and in what areas. For other patients, the therapist may use this section to claim good progress, specify the conditions preventing progress, or assert that while there has been progress the patient has now "plateaued." This may be accompanied by a recommendation to discharge or a suggestion of how to get the patient moving again, such as through the collective pressure of a family conference or consultation with a psychologist. The final section, Plan, has a rather ambiguous status. Some therapists combine it with the Assessment. For example, having a family conference could be part of one's Plan. Some modify the SOAP guidelines somewhat and have a section labeled "Goals and Plans." Others have only a Goals section, sometimes broken into short- and long-range goals, and omit an explicit plan.

Although therapists occasionally discuss what might be included in the various sections of the Progress Note, there is no formal demand for consistency or uniformity. Occasionally a physician may note in team conference that what a therapist has written in the assessment section really belongs in another section. As we shall see later, revisions are sometimes called for if a Progress Note does not support a decision that emerges from the team conference, but this is an individual case matter, not a format issue.

The following is an example of a Progress Note written by a physical therapist. It is taken from the PT section of the Team Conference Notes. Abbreviations used by the therapist in the short progress note are spelled out in the Conference Notes.

Subjective: Patient is easily distracted and agitated. He appears calmer and better able to attend immediately after his friends have left. Attention span is limited to seconds. Patient is disoriented to place and time. He occasionally remembers that he is in a hospital for about 10 minutes.

Objective: Patient exhibits apraxia of extremities. He requires verbal cues with occasional assist for transfers and bed mobility, primarily to sequence the steps of an activity for him. Strength is grossly fair/fair-minus in trunk and extremities. Range of motion appears within normal limits during functional activities except in left lower extremity. Patient stands with knee flexion and plantar flexion left which appear limited by heel cord tightness. Left hip is retracted during stance and trunk is mildly flexed with forward rotation right. Patient ambulates with assistance of one for balance. Weight shift to left is poor, along with balance and posturing as described above. Patient moves rapidly with poor safety techniques. Trunk and extremities are mildly hypnotic. Balance reactions are present, but delayed.

Assessment: Patient is currently limited, primarily by decreased orientation and attention span, as well as apraxia and functional deviations as outlined above.

Goals: Improve orientation and attention span.
> Normalize tone in trunk and extremities and increase strength.
> Increase range of motion, strength, and stability of left lower extremity.
> Improve safety and independence in bed mobility and transfers.
> Improve weight shifting, posture, and gait pattern.
> Assess home and assist with discharge planning when appropriate.

The report from OT generally comes next. In content it overlaps greatly with PT's Notes, particularly in reference to range of motion, strength of muscles, coordination, synergy, spasticity, and patient motivation and orientation. The major differences result from OT's focus on the upper rather than lower part of the body and OT's concern with ADLs, such as dressing and eating, and various homemaking and vocational/avocational skills.

If the patient is being seen in speech therapy, the speech report generally follows. It usually has two sections, one describing problems and one listing goals. Depending on the range of problems discovered in the initial evaluation or during therapy, the speech therapist reports on matters such as tongue and mouth movement, auditory comprehension, memory span, reading speed and comprehension, writing skills, numerical concepts, attention span, and patient orientation, motivation, and insight into problems. Recent progress or regression is noted, sometimes specified with test data, along with comments about how much further improvement can be expected. Following this is a list of goals, such as to improve concentration or reading speed or to decrease perseveration or dysarthria (poor articulation).

The final written Note is presented by a social worker. It describes the strengths and/or weaknesses of the family's support related to the disability. The social worker assesses whether or not the patient is "realistic" about his disability and future and how helpful the family is in providing care and emotional support. Financial concerns are noted here. There also may be comments pertaining to a recent family conference or some mention of when a conference might be scheduled. The last part of the social worker's report usually dwells on the patient's future. There is mention of former employment and whether or not a change in work life will be needed. Vocational or avocational counseling may be recommended. Also included is information on the status of discharge planning. Some patients will return home, others may live with children or relatives, and some will need nursing home placement.

In one or two sentences the social worker also reports on topics labeled "Mental and Emotional Status" and "Vocational/Avocational Status" in the final Team Conference Notes. For the former, the social worker may state simply that the patient is "alert and cooperative" or that he is "confused and disoriented." Assessments of the emotional status of particular family members may be included as are references to a relevant psychological report or plans to have a patient see a psychologist. For the latter topic, the patient's occupation or major daily activity before the onset of the disability is identified, leisure-time interests noted, and any suggestions for vocational or avocational counseling repeated.

The concluding section of the Team Conference Notes, labeled "Reason for Continued Hospitalization" is prepared by a doctor, normally the attending physician. These comments are usually brief, no more than three or four sentences. This section is intended to be a summary of what has preceded, sometimes supplemented with medical information—brief notes on physical disabilities and factors which complicate therapy, such as aphasia, apraxia, personality disturbances, or bowel and bladder problems. For recently admitted patients, a sentence about the patient's potential for improvement in the skills needed for independent living may be included. If a clear view of potential is not yet available for a new patient, it is reported that the specification of problems and goals awaits further evaluation. In forthcoming Notes, however, the team is required to list goals, to show progress toward the goals, and to estimate the continued length of stay.

Progress Note Reviews

Within a day or two of the team conference, Mary W. reviews the Progress Notes submitted on each patient as part of her responsibility as Utilization Review Coordinator. For new patients she checks to see that the therapists feel the patient is a good candidate for rehabilitation, or at least that they state that they expect to conduct further evaluations in order to assess potential and to identify significant problems. In later Progress Notes she checks very carefully for statements about problems, goals, progress, and some estimate of length of stay. The reason for her heightened attention to these matters is that the team alone cannot authorize continued hospitalization beyond the second team conference. A "physician advisor" (reviewer) must agree and certify the decision. The advisors rely on Mary to spot problems for them—problems being any signs of a lack of justification for continued hospitalization.

The utilization review provides the staff at Wilshire with a way to formally document their work and to justify rationally their decisions about continued hospitalization. A primary objective of the review process is to satisfy the PSRO which, through a local health insurer, reviews all claims for payment under Medicare and Medicaid. It is necessary that Wilshire adhere to standards concerning eligibility for admission, quality of care and treatment, and length of stay in order to be fully paid for its services. Since PSRO criteria for utilization review tend to be based on a model of acute care, Wilshire staff are particularly sensitive to how hospitalization is justified—a determination delicately balanced between nursing home, school, and hospital images of the facility and its care. The result has been more denial-of-payment decisions than the staff feel would be justified if more appropriate institutional criteria were applied. Staff's response to the problem has been twofold. First, in cooperation with other comprehensive rehabiliation hospitals in the country, they are working to develop a set of utilization review criteria suitable to physical medicine and rehabilitation. Second, they are attempting formally to convince the local PSRO of the integrity and objectivity of their internal review process in order to gain "delegated" status, in which only a very small sample of Medicare and Medicaid cases is regularly reviewed outside the hospital.

ASSEMBLING ADEQUATE NOTES

Let us now turn to the practice of Progress Note preparation, team conference deliberation, and Progress Note reviews. In this section, we describe how various staff members work to assemble what they believe to be adequate descriptions of progress for individual patients. To describe adequately is to be satisfied that a description conforms to what are believed to be audience understandings or images of that being described.

Therapists work on their Progress Notes throughout the day, whenever they can find time. For some team conferences they may have only one or two Notes to write, which can be completed at a leisurely pace, often in the morning before therapy begins. When they have more patients to report on, note-writing may become a frantic activity. Therapists may work on them during breaks, over lunch, or at the end of the day. Some even complete them at home in the evening or over the weekend.

On one occasion one of us came upon two student OTs in a small room off the OT clinic. They were mulling over the content and wording of their first Progress Note. They tried short descriptive phrases and sentences on scratch paper and then read to one another, frequently asking each other "How does that sound?" and "Do you think that's okay?" Once they had each other's approval, they transferred what they had written onto the clinical Progress Note form and approached their supervising OT for approval. Before handing over the forms, they complained that they had not learned to do this kind of thing in school and admitted to being nervous about reading their notes in front of a physician and other therapists at the forthcoming team conference. The supervisor told them of similar feelings when first starting at Wilshire but assured them that one learns quickly. After the OT supervisor read the Notes, a brief exchange followed:

> *Supervisor:* Looks like a pretty good job but it may be too long. You don't really need to put all the results of the initial evaluation in here. Just say something like "evaluation results in chart." You might want to put a few in, especially if they show a real problem. You also need an assessment and a goal statement—whether you think this patient is a good candidate for rehab and what your goals are for OT. You know, something like that.

> *Student:* How do I know if a patient is a good candidate if the patients' only been here for a couple of days?

> *Supervisor:* Oh...after a while you can size them up pretty fast.

Sometimes it does take time though. If you don't know, just put something like "prognosis depends on further evaluation." That will get you by until you know him a bit better. Why don't you look at some of the other Progress Notes the other OTs have done. You can learn some of the buzz words and how to put things. I think this guy [patient] will be okay. Write an assessment and goal section that sounds positive. He will be here for at least four to six weeks.

Not all Progress Note preparation, of course, is as anxious as this. Some is rather perfunctory and mundane. Therapists sometimes prepare them alone, with little or no interaction with colleagues or patients. They refer to various notes, check test data, and write what might seem, at first blush, to be straightforward accounts of patient progress. Yet regardless of the level of anxiety involved in assembling notes, exchanges like the foregoing one and isolated comments suggest that progress notes attempt to be not just descriptive of facts and activities, but to be *adequately* descriptive. Indeed staff members frequently make pointed references to the appropriate procedure for assembling a suitable description for UR purposes so that it is found adequate.

Objectivity, Subjectivity, and Assessment

Objective data provide one resource for assembling Notes. A wide variety of information is considered to be objective, especially the diagnostic tests administered by the therapists to measure functions such as range of motion, sensation, strength, and capacity for speech and mental tasks, which were described in their practical application in Chapter 3. Also included are ratings of the amount of assistance and supervision needed for various ADLs, such as dressing, eating, walking, wheelchair manipulation, and bodily transfer. Medically related conditions like bowel and bladder problems, skin tone, and extent of and tolerance for pain are also viewed as objective. Since most patients are admitted from other care facilities that have many of the same professional services as Wilshire, outside objective data from speech, OT, PT, and nursing often accompany the patient to Wilshire. While the staff may use this information in part to decide whether or not a patient should be admitted, it does not replace their own diagnostic and evaluative assessments. The utilization review requires in-house (baseline) evaluations soon after the patient arrives, ideally before the first team conference. Testing is needed because the condition of the patient may have changed since the previous evaluation, or measures may not have been taken properly. Up-to-date and accurate information is required to identify current problems, set realistic goals, and measure progress.

Therapists rely on their personal knowledge of the working patient to discover the meaning of objective test data in the service of presenting it as such in relevant sections of their Progress Notes, and they articulate the data with whatever else they know about the patient. When asked why information from other institutions is not relied on for this purpose, a therapist described the important work that goes into making sense of data:

> I guess I could just use the evaluations we get after checking some of them out. You can tell pretty fast if they're way off or not. But I prefer doing my own. That way I can be sure they're accurate and, what's more important, it gives me a chance to get to know the patient. The measures don't tell you that much by themselves. You can't just look at these numbers and say, "Oh, he's the same as somebody else so I can expect him to do this or that." You really have to make the numbers make sense by what else you learn about him. Two patients may look about the same on the tests but are really very different. One can really have a lot more potential then the other, like when you consider their motivation and their desire to perform. It takes time to find out about those kinds of things. I don't take these evaluations all that seriously, at least not right away. After I've worked with a patient for a couple of weeks I can look back and then they make more sense. Then you can see what they are trying to tell you.

The meaning of test data unfolds to therapists as they become acquainted with the patient. In some cases they come to see that the patient is much more skillful than the test data indicate. They may conclude that the patient must have been shy or temporarily confused in the new environment or, while the deficits may in fact have been there, they were of a temporary nature and were quickly overcome with good teaching and hard work. Other patients are thought to be clever enough to hide the severity of their disabilities. The test data then do not reveal the seriousness of the problems. Some are so charming and sociable that they fool the therapist, even on objective indicators. Others are able to perform much better on the tests than in therapy. Of course there are those who, as the therapist reflects, are thought to have shown a close correspondence between test data and actual disability status from the beginning. The point, however, is that only upon reflection is such correspondence, or the lack of it, established.

The initial Progress Note may present a particular challenge to the staff. While in some cases the evaluations have been completed, in other cases the picture is not as clear. Both medical and motivational complications, such as infection or an uncooperative patient, may delay completion of the evaluations. Therapists hesitate to offer an inventory of problems and a plan until the evaluations are finished and they know the patient better. What they sometimes do in such cases is summarize what they have found and note that they expect to complete the evaluations and establish plans and goals by the next team conference, with an explanation of why the data are not yet available. Most therapists are not comfortable with this strategy, however, even though they sometimes use it. Their concern is that they will "look bad" in front of their colleagues in team conference and that third-party payers may raise questions about the delay. In order to avoid embarrassment, therapists sometimes rush through the evaluations during a break in their schedule. Or they may report on the patient's abilities as if they had completed all the evaluations. As one therapist explained, "You can tell pretty well sometimes what they're going to be able to do after a couple of sessions. If you're not sure, you can talk about a lot of other things and no one will notice that you haven't done something yet."

Therapists also account for their lack of objective data in the "objective" section of the SOAP note by virtually "stacking" the "subjective" section. When therapeutically adequate Notes cannot readily be assembled, an educational image of therapy is embellished; description of "subjective" factors, such as motivational and/or learning deficits, then serve as accounts for the lack of objective data or therapeutic results. When results are available—especially appropriate ones—a medical image of patient progress frames the Progress Note; when there is little to report, or what can be reported is unclear or dubious, an educational image tends to predominate. The "S" section of SOAP serves to offset the weaker "O" section.

Even though initial evaluations have been completed, a therapist may still hesitate to fill the Objective section of the first Progress Note when the therapist's overall "feel" for the patient has not crystallized. When the therapist feels that she does not quite see how the patient will fare in rehab over the course of his stay, it is difficult to know how the data are relevant to the particular case. For example, if the therapist feels that a patient may be able to walk again, then standing, balance, coordination, and strength of legs and hips will be important. If, on the other hand, the patient will probably remain in a wheelchair, then other data will be more meaningful. When deciding upon such matters, however, much more is relevant than simply physical skills. As we will discuss more fully later, therapists also consider such matters as patient orientation, motivation, educational level, the family, and future living environment. These other considerations may lead therapists to conclude that while a patient may be able to regain the physical strength needed for walking, disorientation and distractability would make walking dangerous, and thus skills related to wheelchair mobility and safety should be stressed. Or therapists may decide that while the objective evaluations indicate that a patient will probably never be able to walk, they will nevertheless work on walking skills if the patient is so determined to try and is likely to beat the odds.

How do therapists prepare Progress Notes for subsequent team conferences? With the benefit of an additional two weeks of contact with the patient, the therapist is usually able to focus on specific problems and disabilities. Reference to those problems no longer considered relevant to an increasingly crystallized picture of the patient in therapy may be deleted. Other, currently relevant problems identified in initial Progress Notes need only be repeated. For example, in one case an OT had originally reported numerous deficits, including the lack of dressing and feeding skills; two weeks later the patient appeared to be competent in both areas. The therapist admitted that the patient's own efforts had led to improvement, since there had been little teaching in the areas. The therapist suggested that some initial problems were probably the result of "confusion in this new environment" rather then to any real lack of skill. The Notes omitted further mention of feeding deficits but did claim considerable progress in teaching the patient to dress independently. Patient problems were now located in the areas of shoulder and hand strength, homemaking, energy conservation, and avocational interests, and these would provide the goals for further therapy.

Therapists present their Notes in conference as if they were principally describing the patient's concrete condition over time. Once crystallized, what is presented in the Notes has considerable consistency. However, there are factors beyond the patient's progress that make for consistency. One is the therapist's attention to what has been written previously and concern for consistency in subsequent reports. The therapist does not wish to appear contradictory for "no reason at all." Another factor making for consistency is an overall institutional interest in showing progress. When therapists write their initial Progress Note for a patient, they consider areas in which progress can be shown. That seems obvious enough, for their job is to help patients with their disabilities. Yet there is more to the concern than merely what problems show the most promise for rehabilitation. Therapists identify what some of them call "Mickey Mouse" problems in addition to the more serious ones. The problems can be easily evaluated and therapists know that the patient can make progress in the areas. Continued stay can then be readily justified on that basis, if need be, while therapists take their chances working on more difficult disabilities. For example, one patient was recovering the use of the right arm very slowly. The OT felt that at least eight to ten weeks in the hospital would be needed for the patient's confusion to subside and for the arm to regain enough strength and range so that headway could be made in teaching the patient how to use it. In order to justify further stay and to show progress after the patient had shown little improvement over the first two weeks, the therapist started a daily range-of-motion exercise called cone-stacking. This exercise was appropriate for the disability. It was also one where progress could be readily demonstrated. On each subsequent Progress Note the therapist summarized the number of cones the patient could stack and the time it took, and real progress was evident.

Therapists are usually careful to justify their rehab goals by including objective data in Progress Notes. Yet the connection between goals and data is rarely made explicit. There are ordinarily more problems identified in the Objective section of Progress Notes than there are goals following. Goals are often broad enough to include a variety of specific problems. For example, a goal to "improve voluntary control of right lower extremity" covers problems of strength, coordination, and spasticity.

In arriving at goals, therapists consider the subjective status of the patient as well as objective data. Patient motivation and cooperation may be described as being good, poor, or questionable. Mental alertness and responsiveness to verbal or gestural cues are noted. There may be comments on annoying patient characteristics such as crying, whining, or forgetfulness. If the patient complains of pain, this is noted. There may be comments on what the patient hopes to accomplish at Wilshire and how realistic these hopes seem to be. There may also be a comment on the goals, realism, and helpfulness of family members or significant others.

While therapists sometimes find it difficult to distinguish between the subjective and objective information they have about a patient in completing the respective sections of SOAP notes, there is one presentation strategy that universally serves as a distinguishing device. Therapists simply place statements which they attribute to patients in quotes. Quoted statements are sometimes preceded by phrases such as "patient says...," or "patient complains of...." These statements are selected from the assumptions and folklore of, and the many conversations therapists have with, patients. The folklore and conversations ordinarily cover a wide range of topics and may vary considerably in the context of their references to capability, self-confidence, and the future. The therapist selects statements that coincide with other information being presented. If the patient is presented as likely to make good progress, the therapist may include quotes such as: "I'm going to work hard and overcome this thing," or, "Patient states 'I want to go back to work and nothing is going to stop me.'" On the other hand, if the therapist notes that the patient's potential for improvement is questionable, a less hopeful quotation is written into the Note, such as: "Patient complains of being tired of being ordered around. Says, 'I know what's best for me and I'm getting out of here as soon as I can.'" In their separate written styles, the subjective and objective information on Progress Notes serve each other's intended rational purposes—objective data are supported by concrete subjective accounts which, in turn, make the objective data personally meaningful.

Therapists sort through a maze of information and interactions as they decide how best to portray the subjective status of a patient. In the less hopeful case quoted above, for example, the patient had offered numerous compliments to the therapist and, on occasion, was quite positive about progress at Wilshire. The therapist glossed over this, however, dismissing it as irrelevant because, as was explained in conference, the patient was "feigning motivation" and "confabulating a lot." This was not a "true self" speaking. On another occasion, however, when the therapist's attention and interest were focused on the patient's "positive attitude" toward therapy, the now "rare" disgruntled statements were, as the therapist put it, "not showing a truly more serious and optimistic side." To consider such usages contradictory would unjustifiably ignore the ongoing, practical character of description. The subjective status of the patient is presented in writing as part of the particular descriptive task at hand. When therapists themselves take issue with their descriptions—which they sometimes do—the issue (which may center on contradictory usages) also is resolved as part of the particular descriptive business at hand, producing further "contradictions."

Before listing their goals, therapists write an assessment of the patient. As presented, the assessment ostensibly flows from conditions noted in the Objective and Subjective sections of the Note. Given certain physical disabilities and treatment, along with subjective characteristics, a prediction of sorts is made about the likely benefit of further therapy. There are those who, it is written, will obviously benefit, those who will not, and some who are questionable. In practice, however, benefit is calculated against a host of considerations, such as the helpfulness and genuine concern of the family, age, and where the patient will be discharged. The considerations may or may not appear in writing on the Note. When they do, they are presented as objective and subjective clinical facts, conditions of treatment, and response to rehabilitation. When they do not appear, presented clinical justifications for assessments may have little or no resemblance to the reasons entertained in assembling Progress Notes.

Audience Considerations

Audience-related questions concern therapists as they assemble their Notes. Therapists strive to appear thorough, objective, and clinically professional for the purpose of presenting them to both their own colleagues and to any outsiders who may read them. While the Progress Note is formally about the patient and the treatment, because it is presented to a particular audience, what is written receives attention with that audience in mind.

Therapists typically review previous Progress Notes they have written before writing a new one. They offer various reasons for the practice—reasons related to audience considerations. Therapists speak of the need to provide a consistent view of the patient in terms of limitations and problems, progress, and likely future. Themes developed in early Notes should be continued in later ones or, at the very least, changes in them should be clinically justified. For example, if a claim was made in a previous Note that "severe confusion" limits progress in therapy, some reference to this is made in a later one. It may be written that it still limits progress or that the confusion has now subsided. A PT expressed concern for consistency in this way:

> I don't want to look like a fool. It's easy to forget what you wrote the last time because we have so many patients. You need to check to be sure you don't sound like you're talking about another patient, and the report should, how should I say it, sound like it has continuity—like this one should pick up where the last one left off. If

you say that a patient is a great candidate for rehabilitation, then you'd better follow through with a report on progress or explain very carefully what's gone wrong. You know what I'm saying! You write these things so that one thing kind of flows from another. The people who read them expect to see some consistency and you have to remember that when you're writing them up.

While therapists strive for continuity and consistency, they also avoid too much repetition. Another reason then for reviewing previous Notes is to see how things have been said before so that some variation in wording appears in the new Note. Therapists are wary that those who read the Progress Notes might think that they merely copy previous Notes and conclude that they have not put much time or effort into them. For example, in the Subjective section of one Progress Note, an OT described a patient as "highly motivated." In writing the next Note, the therapist mentioned that although the same thing was being said, it was at least presented in a different way by supplying a quotation from the patient ("I'll have to work and exercise real hard"). A speech therapist wrote in one report that the patient's "self-assessment of her limitations is poor." In the next report the description was varied by writing "Patient seems to have little awareness of her deficits"—a variation the therapist made an explicit effort to include.

There is remarkable consistency in the style and language of Progress Notes. Observation of writing practice shows that the consistency is as much a product of staff's effort to present themselves as competent in writing as it is the result of their common concern with being competent in their physical rehabilitation duties. Therapists often discuss with each other what they will write before actually putting pen to paper. Therapists prefer getting "their stories straight" *before* the team conference, where the attending physician and other team members will hear what is read from Progress Notes. As one PT put it:

I don't want to look like an idiot and say the patient is doing very well and can be discharged when OT might say the opposite. So, I check it [the Progress Note] out with OT before. Of course it's not usually that different anyway, but there can be some big goofs sometimes if you don't discuss them first.

Therapists believe that their audiences expect some professional agreement, either in the Progress Notes themselves or in the discussion that takes place in the team conference. The attending physician, for example, needs this in order to write his own commentary. While a physician may not demand consistency in any one conference, he or she is likely to suggest to the therapists who disagree that they do whatever is needed—more tests, a family conference, whatever—to resolve their differences by the next team conference. Therapists hope to avoid being embarrassed by professional contradictions which, on the spur of the moment, are difficult to explain in clinical terms when contradictory comments have already been clinically and professionally documented and presented.

Another audience-related concern is particular physician's receptions of what is read from Notes at the team conference. Some doctors do little more than listen to the Notes as read, perhaps enter the proceedings briefly if a medical issue is raised, and then ask the therapists for an estimate of how much longer the patient should be hospitalized. These team conferences usually move along quickly, with little discussion or debate. Other physicians become more involved. They ask therapists to clarify goals, expand descriptions of progress, or justify recommendations for extended stays. Two physicians particularly are kept in mind when therapists write up their Notes. Keeping them in mind means being wary of the continuity, consistency, and clarity of Progress Notes. In this regard one OT summarized a common sentiment frequently expressed by other staff members:

> I really hate to go to team conferences when she [a female doctor] is there. She can be a real bitch and she's a little crazy, as you saw for yourself. You really have to watch what you say. Sometimes she'll catch you if you can't back up what you say with some data, or if you leave some obvious thing out. Like the other day, I called a patient "disoriented." She made me add to the Note that what I had seen could be called "disorientation." You have to be careful with her and not take so much for granted. She's probably a really good doctor but she doesn't know anything about rehabilitation. Now Dr. Allen, he's different. He's a physiatrist so he knows what he's talking about. You respect the guy. I spend a lot of time on my Notes for him, but it's different being criticized by him than by her. He asks good questions and we have some really good discussions. He'll come down on you too if you haven't written a good Note, but he helps you to make it better. She just makes you feel like a turd.

Therapists are especially meticulous in preparing Progress Notes on patients who have been, or are expected to remain, at Wilshire for unusually long periods of time. They and their supervisors worry that third-party payers may question and fail to remunerate the hospital for lengthy hospitalizations. Therapists are careful to describe in some detail the nature and severity of problems, progress to date, and particularly the goals that justify continued stay. This they collaborate on, both in writing up their Notes before team conferences and in the process of presenting and amending the Notes during the conferences.

THE TEAM CONFERENCE

While some team conferences involve little more than a reading of Progress Notes and a brief summary by the presiding physician, others include extensive discussion and deliberation. Therapists elaborate on what they have written and explain their rationale for selecting particular goals, their evaluations of progress, estimates of length of stay, and similar matters. They frequently comment on issues and questions raised in their respective presentations.

Conference participants' practical knowledge of and concerns for particular patients are considerably more varied and complex than what is written into Progress Notes. As participants fill in what is only sketched in the Note, they reveal a rich interpretative understanding of patients and a rational sense of clinical practice —important dimensions that the written Notes and subsequent revisions and compilations of Notes made available to third parties could not both discursively contain and readily sustain.

Discussing Problems

Patients' problems are a prominent concern of the discussions surrounding Progress Note presentation. Problems are often broader in scope than the specific conditions which resulted in a disability, such as a stroke, and considerably more complex than what can be discovered in the objective data collected and presented by therapists. Typically a problem is anything that interferes with the medical or educational aims of the staff and limits the patient's progress toward independent living.

One frequently mentioned problem is medical complication. As noted previously, some patients are too sick or weak to participate in therapy when they arrive. While the staff try to screen for medical instability, patients may gain admission for "other" reasons. Some patients develop medical problems soon after they have been admitted. For example, infection or pressure sores may develop or worsen. Medical problems keep patients in their rooms, away from therapy. Other medically related problems also interfere with therapy even though the patient is able to attend sessions. For example, if a patient is not making the progress expected by staff, a therapist may suggest to the physician and nurse that this might be due to medications. The patient may be too "drowsy," "lethargic," or "hyperactive." The attending physician may be asked to reduce a dosage or modify a prescription in the hope of increasing the patient's enthusiasm or alertness for therapy.

Pain is another medically related condition that interferes with therapy. A patient may be considered to have the physical strength and skill to perform a certain exercise, but the pain involved limits his ability to actually carry it out. In order to reduce pain, therapists or the physician may suggest some combination of drugs, rest, and special exercises. Complaints of pain are not always accepted at face value, however. Some patients are seen as suffering more from "low pain tolerance" than from real pain. They are called "complainers," "bitchers," or "cry babies." The relevant sections of Progress Notes indicate problems with motivation or orientation rather than with limitations resulting from real pain. In this regard, consider the following brief exchange between a physician and a PT during the team conference. The doctor asks the therapist about written comments concerning the patient's poor motivation and lack of follow-through:

Dr.: I agree that we haven't seen much progress in the past two weeks, but I thought the problem was the pain in her back and legs. When I talk to her, she seems quite motivated to me.

PT: She may have a little pain there but it's no big deal. She can do it if she wants to but she's such a big cry baby. She likes everyone to do for her and feel sorry for her. She just lies in bed and moans when she tries the exercises. Everyone on the North Court hears her and says, "Poor Betty, poor Betty."

Dr.: So what do we do?

PT: Just get tough with her. Make her do the exercises no matter how loud she cries.

[*Others in attendance agree that the pain is not as great as the patient claims and that she should be dealt with more firmly.*]

Accepting a bodily problem as medical is not a straightforward matter of accurately reading its symptoms. Symptoms, such as pain, are always subject to the immediate and ongoing interests and related understandings of those who interpret them, which, in turn, inform responses to symptoms. While this may be evident in staff deliberations, it does not appear in writing.

Problems are also located in the motivation or emotional status of patients. Therapists depend upon the patient's own desire to live as independently as possible and attempt to strengthen the desire as they work with patients. Patients who are seen as striving for less may be scorned for taking up space in the hospital. Such patients are recognized through a variety of clues. Therapists take note of what patients say about their goals for therapy and their desired futures. They also consider complaints and gripes as evidence of emotional status. Patients who have goals that are less ambitious than their condition warrants, or than a facility like Wilshire aspires to, are viewed as posing motivational barriers to therapy. These barriers may be even more formidable if accompanied by emotional difficulties. A therapist may include a quotation from a patient in describing his motivation. Or the therapist may simply write and report that the patient is highly motivated, unmotivated, uncooperative, or something similar. In many cases, descriptions that are read pass with little comment because other participants at the team conference are able to fit what is said with what they know about the particular patient or the typical patient. On occasion questions are raised about what motivational or emotional problems cited mean in a particular case. In their discussion, participants both rationally and empirically "fill-in" the meaning of problems only sketched or listed in the Progress Note (Buckholdt and Gubrium, 1979a). They use their diverse experiences with the patient as resources to explain why they have cast him or her in a particular way, and they fit their experiences together in a reasonable and consistent way. Those who later read the Notes will similarly make sense of what is sketched in them, not necessarily bringing to bear the same experiences and reason. Each discussion of problems noted may serve to interpret them differently.

Therapists call on their personal knowledge of the working patient in support of their written comments. For example, consider the response of a physical therapist who was asked about a patient's subjective status by a doctor substituting for a colleague on vacation.

> *Dr.:* I noted in this and the last Note that you don't feel this patient is a very good bet for further improvement. I've talked with her and she seems aware of her problems and I thought she wanted to help herself. I thought we had a pretty good record with MS [multiple sclerosis] patients.

PT: We do but I don't think she'll go very far. She gives you that motivated stuff when she thinks we are getting fed up and may send her home. She's really an institutional type.

Dr.: What do you mean?

PT: She likes to be around and be taken care of. She comes to therapy just enough to keep me from really getting angry. She'll come for several days in a row and then says she's too tired.

Dr.: But that's one of the problems with MS. Stamina really varies from day to day.

PT: I know, but in her case it's more than stamina. She's really lost whatever drive she might have had to help herself.

Dr.: Well...you know her better than I do. I was just curious why you wrote that in the note.

A few patients are described as being uncooperative because they are overresponsive or too independent. The ideal patient is one who desires independence but who, at the same time, dutifully follows the directions of the therapists while in the hospital. As therapists talk about patients in team conferences, it is clear that this type of patient is particularly perplexing. On occasion they are admired; at other times they are found annoying. The patients sometimes claim that the only way they can improve is to get out of the hospital. They may invent their own exercises and may skip therapy in order to exercise on their own. While therapists appreciate initiative, they feel that such patients are unwise to ignore professional instruction. Annoyance sometimes turns to hostility as therapist and patient engage in an escalating series of mutual accusations. In team conferences therapists recount their encounters with such patients in the service of explaining what lies behind denotations of "uncooperative" or "hostile."

Therapists also consider the patient's mental status as they elaborate on their Progress Notes. They expand on the logic that leads them to conclude that a patient's mental condition bodes well or ill for progress in therapy. Intelligence and level of education are sometimes part of the overall picture. If a patient seems to be "smart" or has a graduate degree, for example, they may use this as a basis for concluding that he has the mental "tools" to take advantage of rehabilitation. Sometimes a patient's former employment provides a clue on ability to learn; a dentist's potential, for example, is compared favorably with a bus driver's. Indeed, taken alone, a professional background is an implicit sign for therapists of acuity. Beyond intelligence, education, and employment, therapists also speak of the patient's "orientation," "confusion," and "insight." These, too, are aspects of the patient's current mental status and are believed to have a significant effect on intelligence, to "make a difference" in how the patient's background is evaluated. For example, an OT argued that while a business executive had no doubt been very successful vocationally, progress at Wilshire was impeded by "severe confusion" and an inability to follow directions. Patients who show insight, on the other hand, are those who understand both what has happened to them and the significance of their problems. They are thought to be good candidates for rehabilitation.

Considering Presented Goals and Progress

Talk about patient problems in team conferences is accompanied by discussion of how much progress a patient can be expected to make or has made, a question whose answer underpins recommendations for continued hospitalization. A patient's medical condition, motivation, mental status, insight, and other factors, such as the concern of his family, are brought to bear in considerations of likely or achieved progress. While therapists may have their own personal and professional reasons for wanting to help patients, their concern for progress in the utilization review significantly centers on third-party expectations. In Chapter 3 we discussed the practical process of linking standards of progress with concrete performances and the interpretation of the meaning of standards by therapists. In this section we expand the discussion of the interpretation of progress by describing how it enters into related team conference proceedings.

Progress Notes commonly contain information on progress in therapy. Sometimes it appears in the form of objective data on such matters as strength, range of motion, or standing tolerance, or in the form of ratings of the amount of assistance required for an activity. At other times the Notes are more general, stating simply that a patient has, say, "improved greatly" or "hasn't improved much" in one or more areas.

As they read their written Notes in team conference, therapists typically stop to elaborate what they have written. They may relate progress or its absence to emotional or mental states. They may even base their assessment of progress on these states. For example, one therapist admitted that judgment of recent gains was based much more on an improvement in motivation than on any real change in physical skill. Because of confidence that improvement in physical functioning would soon be evident, the therapist reported it as gain. The reverse also occurs: therapists predict regression or a slowing of progress because of changes in emotional or mental status.

An important consideration is whether or not goals as written are significant enough for a place like Wilshire. Consider, for example, a situation in which PT and OT admitted having a difficult time arriving at goal statements for an elderly female patient who had suffered a stroke. They liked her and wanted her to stay for treatment, but they weren't sure what physical or mental functions she would recover or whether she would return home or be transferred to a nursing home. By the second team conference, they had adopted several goals and were able to report some progress. As stated, the goals were quite general, focused on increasing the strength and range of motion in arms and legs. While such goals are not all that unusual, the presiding physician took the opportunity to lecture therapists on the kinds of goals selected. As the doctor explained,

> We really have to be careful about vague goals like these. Ask yourself, "Are they really appropriate for a place like Wilshire?" Maybe if a person isn't able to be more independent when they leave we shouldn't admit them in the first place. I see high-level goals as returning a person to pretty much the same state they were in before or at least making them as independent as possible. While strength and mobility are important, they're not the same thing as doing for yourself. We also have to be careful getting too close to the patient. We lose objectivity, and may see progress when it isn't there—we get to know the patient better and then it seems like change has really occurred somehow, even if it's very little.

While staff members agonize over the difficult issues of whether or not progress has occurred and whether gains are being made in areas that are clinically important for the long-range welfare of the patient, such doubts only temporarily disturb the team conference's presentational concerns. Attention soon focuses on the issue of how to write up goals and report progress. The physician whom we quoted above, for example, soon prods therapists to "come up with goals," start "measuring progress," and "put it down in black and white" after they had discussed the problems they were having in doing so. Issues of valid measurement and the significance of goals are pushed aside in the press of satisfying the standard appearance of the utilization review, which tacitly requires goals and assessments of progress to be adequately presented in writing for third-party review.

When therapists report gains in patients who made little headway before coming to Wilshire, they take much of the credit. When the reverse occurs and patients who were reported to have made good progress before coming to Wilshire now seem to be moving slowly, if at all, staff members look for other explanations. In one case the staff was somewhat distressed over a patient, Steve Lester, who seemed to be making little progress at Wilshire because of his "extreme confusion and disorientation," but who had been reported by the acute care hospital in which he had been a patient to have made rapid gains and to be a very sociable and likeable fellow. His wife corroborated the gains and complained that he appeared to change, "as if a spell had been cast over him," en route to Wilshire. In accounting for the change in the team conference, a nurse suggested that the wife and hospital personnel may have lied in order to get him admitted to Wilshire. The physician discounted this explanation because he knew the people at the other hospital and felt that they would not try to deceive him. Other possibilities were suggested until the physician remembered that the wife had told him that her husband was honored by having had a "Steve Lester Day" when he was discharged from the other hospital. Almost the entire staff of the small hospital attended the party. The physician used this event to argue that Steve had been the "pet" of the hospital and that he had probably "withdrawn" and "regressed" when he could not assume the same role at Wilshire. He added that the role of hospital favorite probably misled the staff into seeing many more gains than were actually present. In another case, a female patient who had suffered a stroke was said to be making little progress walking without maximal assistance. The therapists were concerned about how this would look to the insurance company since the acute care hosptial from which she was transferred reported that she could walk independently. The physician eased their concerns by asking, "But what do they mean by walking? She might take a step or two by herself but that's not walking, in my book." He promised to say something about this in his summary.

Progress is a frequent theme of conversations between staff and patients or family members. Sometimes staff initiate talk about progress with the intent of motivating, reinforcing, or warning patients. Patients often ask how they are doing and family members ask for progress reports. On occasion there are disagreements over how much progress has been made and the evidence used to support one estimate or another. Although these disagreements are not recorded in Progress Notes, staff members sometimes do refer to them in team conference and attempt to justify their own view that either more or less progress can be claimed.

Some patients and family members cannot see the progress claimed by therapists. They feel that there has been little if any improvement. One common explanation used by the therapists to resolve the difference of opinion is to suggest that the patient or family member is gauging progress with an inappropriate set of criteria; they are comparing the patient with what he or she was like before the accident or onset of illness. Rather, they should contrast current status with the patient's condition shortly after the disabling incident. Disagreements can also arise at the other end of the spectrum when patients, and particularly family members, claim more progress than staff are willing to certify. Sometimes these disagreements are traced to the kind of patient who "makes you think more progress has been made than is the actual case." Staff sometimes caution one another in team conference to be wary of patients who are "unnaturally cheerful" or who have a "bubbly exterior." Appearances may hide real deficits and minimal progress.

Patients and family members can also be mistaken in what they use as evidence for progress. One female patient, for example, had no functional speech, according to the speech therapist. The family reported, however, that when they took her to a restaurant one Sunday, she ordered "roast beef and mashed potatoes." The staff concluded that this, if it did indeed happen, was involuntary, habitual speech, and thus not functional. In another case a family reported that a patient had been able to play poker while on a home visit. The family wondered if this could be seen as improvement in cognitive functioning. The speech therapist considered the possibility but concluded that the area of the brain that, as the therapist put it, "controls numbers," probably was not affected by the stroke in the first place so this should not be seen as an improvement in cognitive capacity.

Sometimes, however, family members or patients are successful in convincing staff that more progress has taken place than staff members realize. One patient came to be seen by staff members as being particularly hopeless. He had been stricken by a disabling virus while on an airplane; he had boarded the plane as a normal person and emerged almost completely paralyzed. He had been in a hospital on the East Coast for several weeks before coming to Wilshire. The staff worked intensively with him for several weeks but they became discouraged when they saw little if any gain. The wife, who visited daily, eventually convinced them that progress was indeed occurring. Staff's problem was that they had not seen what he was like before coming to Wilshire. In another instance, therapists were prepared to discharge an elderly female patient after two weeks at Wilshire because of lack of progress in therapy. Her son, an educational psychologist, objected. On methodological grounds, he argued that they had selected unreasonable goals for a woman of her age and that, given a more relevant plan for treatment, progress could indeed be shown. Although not totally convinced by the argument, staff members agreed in team conference that some progress had indeed occurred and that they would keep her for at least four more weeks.

Considering the Patient's Future

Considerations of the future touch on various aspects of the patient's hospital life. How will the patient spend his or her time after discharge? The person who plans on returning to work, for example, may pose a somewhat different sent of contingencies for therapists than one who will stay home. When it is learned that a banker plans to retire in the near future, therapists take this into account in planning therapy. In one case, the goals for therapy were altered in conference when the staff learned that a middle-aged woman who had been a housewife and homemaker planned to work for the first time in two decades. Staff weren't convinced that she could find employment, but the knowledge of her seeking it altered their therapeutic considerations with a view toward a future worklife. The speech therapist, for one, expanded testing and teaching beyond the elementary cognitive and functional language skills needed around the home and included some attention to "higher level cognitive and communication skills."

The presence and willingness of others who can assist the patient after discharge also enters into future considerations. These others are often family members. While the hospital goal is for the patient to be as independent as possible, in practice the optimum attainment of this goal is interpreted against a background of whatever is known about the patient, the family, and significant others. A patient who has "real" family poses a different set of problems and possibilities than a similarly disabled person who has none. This became apparent in a number of situations where the future living arrangements of a patient changed unexpectedly and therapists modified their rehab plans. Once staff learned that a brother and a concerned neighbor would, several times each day, look in on an elderly female patient who lived alone and prepare her meals, the staff decided that her problems were actually less severe than they originally thought. In another case, the staff decided that they needed to delay the discharge of a middle-aged patient suffering from MS when they learned that her daughter, who had been assisting her mother with household chores, would be leaving home. To justify her unexpected stay, the patient's problems were written up as more severe and her past progress as somewhat less than satisfactory.

The mere availability of assistance is not the only consideration in discharge planning. Those who are to assist are expected to be competent and concerned. If help is thought likely to be haphazard or selfish, its value diminishes. The availability and the intent to make use of continuing professional rehabilitative services is also relevant to therapists. For example, if a patient will enter a nursing home which is thought to have good PT and OT departments, therapists evaluate problems and progress at Wilshire in light of the continuing treatment. What might be seen as a serious enough deficit to justify continued hospitalization at Wilshire becomes less of a problem when a patient decides to enter a good nursing home or expects to continue rehab on an outpatient basis. The rehab problems of a male stroke victim were judged to be less severe then originally thought when staff learned in team conference that his daughter was an occupational therapist; in the light of this, his wife's request that he be released within a week or two seemed more reasonable. In contrast, another patient was kept longer then originally anticipated because staff felt that even though the spouse had attended therapy sessions regularly and knew how to assist and teach, they lived in a remote rural region of the state and probably would not have access to good outpatient services.

From Initial Write-up to Final Submission

Team conference participants not only consider and discuss what has been written up as Progress Notes by individual team members and presented in the conference; they also deliberate over how individual Notes sound in the light of newly found problems and information and how they fit together for presentation in writing to third parties. The final written report, the "Team Conference Notes," is considered to be an overall clinical assessment of the patient's rehab status by his team based on Progress Notes, not an aggregate of individual reports and understandings of treatments and responses. Thus at one or more points during most team conferences, attention shifts from the facts of a case as written in Progress Notes and discussed by participants to how "things should be put now" for the Conference Notes. Sometimes the shift is subtle and momentary. A physician may briefly interrupt proceedings to ask a therapist to include in a Progress Note information that has just surfaced in discussion. At other times the shift is marked and sustained. Conference participants focus their discussion on what they need to report in order to justify whatever it is they have decided about a patient. The shift in attention is accompanied by a shift in concern, from the consistency and reasonableness of Progress Notes to their substantive adequacy—the latter being a focused, third-party consideration.

In their concern for adequacy, physicians sometimes suggest that therapists add more detail to their reports if a case looks like it may be a difficult one. They may ask that Progress Notes be "beefed-up" so that the hospital can show why an unusually long stay is warranted. There are a variety of reasons for why estimating length of stay is considered difficult. Therapists complain to each other about the problem of not knowing how much return of function to expect in a recent stroke victim. Patient's with apraxia are hard to evaluate as are uncooperative or combative patients. Ambiguity about the patient's own goals for the future, living arrangements following discharge, the helpfulness of the family, or possible psychological problems may complicate therapeutic planning.

Sometimes therapists are simply not able to complete their evaluations, particularly before the first team conference, because of vacation days, unexpected problems with the patients, or an unusual amount of time spent in other team conferences. If the therapists, particularly PT and OT, are not prepared to suggest a time frame for discharge by the first, and sometimes the second, team conference, the physician usually reluctantly agrees to wait. It is understood, however, that the therapists will supply a written explanation of why a case is a difficult one, an explanation that centers on the patient and *his* or *her* problems. One physician offered this suggestion to a PT:

> I can see how he'd be hard to test. Apraxia like that makes it hard to know what he can do. He may just pop out of it in a day or two or it may last for weeks. Why don't you say some more about it in your Note. That way if we need to keep him longer than normal, we can show the reasons later on. We don't want to make it look like it's no big deal now and then change our minds later on.

A PT foresees the same concern when describing a strategy in preparing initial Progress Notes in difficult cases:

> With some of them it's really hard to know how much progress
> they'll make. Sometimes I can't say. How can I estimate the time
> after a week or so? So I put in stuff that I know from the evaluation,
> nitty-gritty stuff like range of motion and assistance. I also talk
> about other things, like his attitude or motivation, that kind of
> thing. You have to let them know that you know the patient and
> that there are real problems. But you have to be careful that you
> don't get carried away and make them look too bad or too hopeless.
> The insurance company might ask why they were ever admitted
> if they're hopeless.

Therapists are well aware of the fact that the average stay at
Wilshire is monitored by the local PSRO and that the hospital
intends to keep this average at an acceptable 38 days. Thus they
routinely estimate a four-to-six week hospital stay unless they
feel that special considerations can justify a longer stay, say,
six to eight weeks or more. The physician typically accepts the
routine recommendation unless he feels there are special medical
reasons for pushing back the date. For example, one physician
suggested that a recently discovered infection may interrupt therapy so they probably should estimate eight weeks rather than the
six suggested by the therapists. If the physician suspects a possibility of retroactive nonpayment, the expected length of stay is
shortened. Citing knowledge of a previous case like the one before
him, where payment was denied, a physician recommends six
weeks rather than the proposed eight, adding that if more time is
required, they can work on justifying it later.

Once the length of stay is estimated, team members use the
estimate in future Notes as they establish both the rationale for
and the accuracy of their initial estimate. When the time comes in
a team conference to summarize the Progress Notes presented by
the therapists and to estimate continued lengths of stay, the physician invariably considers previous Notes and estimates. The estimate for continued stay usually comes easily, as the physician
concludes something like, "Let's see, last time we said six weeks so
now [two weeks later] it's four weeks. Is that okay with everybody?"
Heads typically nod in agreement. There are occasional side comments, accompanied by chuckles, about "how scientific we are."
More commonly the next case is quickly taken up.

Sometimes, however, issue is taken with the strategy of simply
reducing the previous estimate by two weeks. Someone may feel
that a patient should be discharged sooner than was projected.
But, at the same time, there is the concern that the insurance

company may decide, in retrospect, that the patient should not have been admitted in the first place if the stay is too short. A therapist or doctor may suggest that a patient be kept a week longer than originally recommended so that "it won't look funny to the insurance company." On one occasion, a physician considered such a suggestion and then rejected it, explaining, "we need some short stuff like this to lower our overall average [length of stay]." In most cases where the original estimate is revised, however, a longer stay is suggested.

In deliberation over how to put things in writing, staff constantly weigh their own ongoing evaluations of a case against how what they present on paper will be evaluated by third parties who later pay for their services. Whatever their knowledge of third-party payment details, all staff members make references to, and are wary of—in big-brother fashion—the "insurance companies."

Medical problems complicate continued hospitalization decisions and their justification. The staff attempt to deny admission to the medically unstable. Occasionally they are admitted and then create accountability problems. For example, several patients had serious heart problems and their therapists worried continually that they would have an attack during exercise. More common, however, are medical problems that arise after admission. Some of the more frequent medical complications are urinary tract infections, bed sores, and various respiratory ailments.

If the medical problem is seen as serious and/or long term, the staff generally do not hesitate to recommend discharge to an acute care hospital. This decision is justified in part because Wilshire does not have the facilities to handle many types of serious cases. In case of an emergency such as heart attack, they do what they can until a paramedic unit arrives and transports the patient to an acute care hospital. A second reason for discharging a patient with serious medical problems to an acute care hospital is that third-party payers may refuse payment if it is apparent that the patient is not well enough to benefit from rehabilitative therapy. While staff recognize this possibility and often recommend discharge for such patients, they do not always approve of the required decision. In many instances they feel that they could provide much better care and supervision than the patient will receive in the acute care hospital, given that a primary nurse at Wilshire looks after a maximum of four patients. For example, they had no doubt about their superior capability for treating a patient with pneumonia. They also feel that the insurance company is very shortsighted in these cases, for the basic charges at Wilshire are about $225 per day while comparable care in an acute hospital is much more costly.

When medical complications are less serious, the staff face a dilemma. Should they discharge a patient or keep him and treat the problem themselves? In many instances they believe that they can provide effective short-term treatment. They try to avoid discharging and then readmitting because of the inconvenience to the patient and to themselves. Each admission requires a complete reevaluation of the patient, and the movement back and forth may slow the patient's momentum in rehabilitation. On the other hand, the hospital also risks denial of payment.

These unforeseen issues are discussed in team conference before Progress Notes are considered to be ready for submission. Therapists report that medical problems and their side effects, such as pain, are interferring with therapy. A patient may miss several sessions, or if he does attend, little is accomplished. The physician and therapists discuss what to do. They may consider how much progress has been made to this point and whether the medical problem is a real hindrance to therapy or the patient is merely using it as an excuse to avoid therapy. They may decide to discharge the patient or, more typically in nonlife-threatening situations, to keep him or her for a week to see if they can clear up the problem and then resume therapy. When the latter decision is made, the issue becomes "how to put it" in Progress Notes. In some cases the doctor merely tells the therapists that the attending physician will "take care" of the descriptive problem in the section of the final Team Conference Notes labeled "Reason for Continued Hospitalization." The physician may reassure the therapists by saying something like "Don't worry, I'll word this one carefully" or "I'll take a little extra time writing this one up." Some physicians consult therapists about what they should say. Consider, for example, the following conversation concerning a patient with a bladder infection that has kept her away from therapy for a week:

Dr.: So there are some signs that this bladder thing is clearing up. Another couple of days and she should be back in therapy? I don't think we really need to discharge her. After all, she was making good progress before this thing hit. I'll be careful to say the right thing. We have some time. Are there any suggestions?

PT: She is really motivated and has been upset about missing therapy.

OT: We can always work on some other goals until she's up and about. Like we can...

Dr.: Good, I'll be sure to mention that her motivation is good and that we still have some goals to work on... [*Turning to OT*] What would you do, range work in the upper extremities?

OT: Right. Strengthening too.

Speech Therapist: Why not say that we're using this time to consolidate our gains so that we can make even better progress once the problem clears up?

Dr.: Marvelous! That'll make it look like we're not just sitting on our hands until she gets better.

[*At this point the physician turns to the observer and comments about feeling a lack of formal training in dealing with "creeping" and "know-it-all" bureaucracies like the PSRO, suggesting that it is difficult to translate good medical decision-making into a form that will be acceptable to outside reviewers. The physician also mentions, though, that with practice, wording of reports has improved so that claims for payment are less likely to be rejected.*]

In most cases where nonlife-threatening medical problems interfere with progress in therapy, the physician and the therapists come to some agreement about goals that can be pursued until the problems are corrected. The patient can stay at Wilshire unless the problem persists for what is vaguely perceived as an unreasonable length of time. Unreasonableness is partly defined in terms of what the PSRO is likely to object to, and this, in turn, depends in part on how skillfully the staff are able to word their Notes. Of course "unreasonableness" also has a therapeutic criterion in how much interference with therapy therapists can tolerate before they begin to feel that the patient should be discharged. Amount of interference is not calculated according to some precise standard or set of guidelines. Like considerations of other patient performances, the judgment depends on a number of factors, including past progress of the patient, motivation, cooperation, charm of personality, and the helpfulness and optimism of family. On the other hand, medical problems are sometimes used as a basis for discharging objectionable patients who, if they had been more cooperative and helpful, might have remained hospitalized. According to staff, in addition to providing a convenient way of "getting rid of" someone, discharges for medical complications are useful in presenting the staff as conscientiously conducting its internal review on the basis of rehabilitation criteria.

While rehabilitation ideally is both staff's chief therapeutic and descriptive concern, one physician frequently challenged the importance of therapists' work in contrast to that of medical care. These challenges were marked by supercilious charges of therapeutic staff's ignorance in medical matters, charges which were frequently abrasive. Most of the therapists disliked this physician, believing that admissions and hospitalizations of patients who were medically interesting but had little hope of benefiting from PT or OT occurred at this physician's instigation. The normally quiet tension between the medical interests of supervising physicians and the rehabilitation interests and descriptive needs of therapists came to a head during a team conference when a few therapists recommended a discharge date different from that of the doctor. In the following exchange the physician reacts negatively to the suggestion that the patient should be discharged in one more week, due to lack of progress in treatment and the difficulties of justifying continued hospitalization:

Dr.: You PTs and OTs think you have the only important work to do here. Well, you're wrong! What you do is important but the medical condition of the patient is just as important and that's my concern. This patient has some problems that you know nothing about. If we can clear those up, he'll make good progress in your PT. I want him kept for a while longer so please find some goals you can work on.

PT: We may not get paid if we keep him.

Dr.: You let me worry about that. Just find something to work on. I know you can, you always do in other cases. I know how to word these things if I have to. If you want me to, I can even overdocument progress. We've shown progress in our other reports and we can do it again.

At some point in each patient's stay, staff decide on a discharge date. The formal process by which this is accomplished is built around PSRO criteria. Goals and progress are reviewed no later than ten days after admission, every two weeks thereafter, and sometimes weekly if there are serious questions about continued stay. An estimate is made at each team conference about continued length of stay, based on how much progress is being made toward goals set for therapy and bounded by a set of guidelines stipulating that most patients will stay four to six weeks, while some may require six to eight weeks or longer if they have more serious problems and continued progress can be shown. Although goals and progress certainly are important when staff consider discharge, other, formally hidden, considerations also enter their decision-making. These do not appear in writing in the same way they are encountered in practice.

One factor that staff consider in deciding upon a discharge

date is what has been said in prior reports, with an attempt to adhere to original estimates. While the estimates are ostensibly based on the problems and progress of patients, in practice they also depend on what outside reviewers are thought to expect. Staff may admit to each other that initial estimates were wrong, that the patient could benefit from additional therapy, or, on the contrary, that he or she could be discharged earlier. Yet they tend to adhere to the original plan in the service of statistical and deliberative rationality. Of course circumstances arise which require that initial estimates be modified, together with ways of justifying changes.

Another factor affecting discharge planning is disagreements among team conference participants. Although they usually resolve differences of opinion before team conference, occasionally disputes arise during the proceedings. There may be disagreement over whether a patient should have been admitted in the first place. In one case, for example, a nurse argued that the patient "has no reason for being in a place like this." The PT, however, saw some potential for progress and had identified what were described as "attainable goals." The doctor told the nurse that the patient would stay and that the nurse should not complain since the patient would be easy to take care of. The nurse agreed with this latter point, adding that there actually would be no problem since the Progress Note had not yet been written.

A more common disagreement occurs over the patient's ability to benefit from further hospitalization. One therapist may feel that important, beneficial skills can be taught, while another argues that little more can be done. For example, at a prior team conference, the staff concluded that the patient could stay two more weeks and then would be discharged. However, at what was to be the final team conference, the OT reported that some "unexpected gains" had been made over the past two weeks and requested more time to work on homemaking, work simplification, and safety skills. The therapist suggested that the woman could be more independent at home than they had anticipated. The physician then asked the other team members what they thought:

> *Social Worker:* I'm sure the husband won't mind if she stays. He wants her to be as independent as possible.
>
> *Speech Therapist:* I don't really need to see her any more. She's doing fine.
>
> *Dr.:* We can keep her without speech, but we really need to have PT. What do you say?

PT: Okay with me. I can always find something. We can keep her for two more weeks.

Dr.: Well, I think we can justify two more weeks then if it's alright with everybody.

Disagreements are not always resolved so easily, or with this result. Some patients are discharged even though one or more therapists feel that further rehab is justified. If a therapist objects to continued stay in part because the patient is personally objectionable, he or she may argue for discharge more forcefully. Whatever the nature of disagreements or intensity of debate, however, team conference participants strive to make their conclusions reasonable as they describe the patient in Progress Notes, which often means that Notes must be revised or rewritten before final submission to the secretary who compiles the Team Conference Notes.

Another challenge to discharge planning and its justification comes from unexpected developments in what is foreseen as the patient's life following discharge. In considering discharge, the staff assess the patient's likely destination in terms of maintenance of goals achieved at Wilshire, continued development, and availability of assistance in activities of daily living. Social workers have the primary responsibility for seeing that the postdischarge environment is suitable. They counsel family members, persuade them to attend therapy sessions, schedule family conferences, arrange for outpatient therapy, contact the Visiting Nurses Association and the Division of Vocational Services, and arrange for nursing home placement, among other discharge details.

While discharge planning begins soon after the patient enters the hospital, unexpected turns of events in the post-discharge environment complicate discharge planning. For example, a daughter decides not to move in with her disabled mother after all, or a wife decides that her husband is too big for her to handle and that he might have to be placed in a nursing home. Or a wife prizes her new-found independence, discovered during her husband's hospitalization and does not want him back in the home. In another instance, at his wife's behest, a son decides that his mother would interfere too much with his family life and wants time to work out a living arrangement for the mother with one of his brothers or sisters. In cases where unexpected developments are less serious challenges to discharge planning and justification, they are, nonetheless, taken into consideration in what is finally written into Progress and Team Conference Notes. For example, one family had planned to take their summer vacation when their grandmother was to be discharged, and the hospital had to justify an additional two week stay for her. In another case a son refused to accept his mother into his home until his own son returned from a hospital where he was being treated for pneumonia.

Such problems are not always family-related. An appropriate nursing home may be full and thus not able to accept a patient considered to be ready for discharge from Wilshire; or a nursing home may reverse an acceptance because it is felt the patient requires too much care. Arranging a new placement may at some times take several weeks. In other instances, delays in discharge are more related to internal than to external scheduling issues. A social worker, for example, may go on vacation before completing final discharge plans; or a therapist becomes ill and is unavailable to complete a final evaluation or report.

When a patient is to be hospitalized longer than anticipated, the change is justified. Sometimes it is decided that two more weeks "are needed," without attention being called to the fact that this is two weeks beyond what was initially specified. At other times the change is reported to be the result of a change in the patient's rehab status, whether objective or subjective. Unjustifiable reasons are not revealed in writing.

Continued hospitalization requires treatment goals. When there are no longer any goals, the patient is discharged. Therapists are reminded of this as they write their Progress Notes, and this is of special concern when they know that a change in discharge date is likely. If a therapist fails to consider an expected delay, or learns of a change in discharge plans at the team conference, she is routinely asked to add to, amend, or even rewrite Progress Notes in light of the change. Consider the following exchange which takes place after conference participants are informed by the social worker that a nursing home will unexpectedly be unable to accept a patient for at least ten days.

> *PT:* That's okay with me. She's nice enough. But I've met all my goals and my "evals" are done.

> *Dr.:* You're all going to have to look at your Notes and find some more goals. You can all find something to work on for a while; use your imaginations. By the way, you don't have to do the final evaluations over. Just move the date back.

> *PT:* I'll look over some earlier Notes. I think I remember some problems that I really haven't worked on that much. We can always

give her more gait training if nothing else. She's still a little uncertain going up and down steps.

[Other therapists now enter the conversation and discuss what they will work on. Each of them agrees to identify additional problems and specify goals.]

Progress Notes that are completed before it is learned that discharge plans now require writing new ones are usually either revised or destroyed. The opportunity to compare old and new versions of Progress Notes that result from changes in discharge plans is rarely available. On one occasion, however, we had the opportunity to observe directly the creation of a new Note for "unjustifiable" reasons and to compare the old with the new. Conference participants had just agreed that there was little more they could do for a patient, that no further goals could be set, and that the patient was a good candidate for a nursing home placement. It was concluded that discharge be completed within the week. The social worker promised to arrange a final family conference but then noted that there would be a delay. A son wanted to be involved in the discharge and transfer but was going on vacation for two weeks. The physician then suggested that the therapists would need to reconsider what they had written in their Progress Notes, reminding them that they must have goals and show progress if the patient is to stay for two more weeks. The physician avoided telling them what to write but did make it clear that some sort of revision would be needed if continued stay "would pass inspection later on." At this point several participants suggested that they could find some things to work on, like transfers and upper-extremity powerbuilding. The PT actually wrote a new Progress Note while others were talking and then tore up the old one and threw it away. At the conclusion of the team conference, one of us retrieved the old note. The old note read as follows (explanations of abbreviations added):

S—[*Subjective*]: Pt. [patient] lives on 2nd floor—this is *not* feasible for the patient. c/o [complains of] pain in the low back.

O—[*Objective*]: Pt. is ambulating in the parallel bars approx. 30 pt. [per trial] (ambulation is preceded by HP [hot pack] to the low back) Pt. puts 1/2 of his wt. or more on the Ⓛ LE [left lower extremity]. In the stance phase he cannot push up c̄ [with] his arms to partial wt. bear on the Ⓛ LE. Mat activities c̄ the LEs are good. Ⓛ hip F: R hip G. Pt. can tolerate 1/2 hour exercises.

A—[*Assessment*]: Try to contact Dr. Smith, his orthopedic surgeon.

P—[*Plan*]: Cont [continue] on present program.

Goals: Depends on whether doctor will change his orders.

In the revised note, the PT copied the subjective and objective sections from the original, adding "not always alert, often confused" to the Subjective portion. The following sections were altered, however, with an explicit statement of goals, now included in the Assessment section. The Assessment and Plan portions of the note then read this way:

A—[*Assessment*] Goals: ↑[increase] VC [vital capacity], ↑ambulation endurance, ↑safety

P—[*Plan*]: Recommend nursing home placement.

While staff members routinely consider the expections of third-party payers as they prepare Progress Notes, attention to this audience is more explicit in some circumstances than in others. When plans for discharge must be altered, often for reasons unrelated to the patient's clinical status at Wilshire, staff face the problem of justifying continued hospitalization. As one physician put it, "You have to not only help the patient and the family and be sensitive to their needs, you also have to cover your own behind."

REVIEWING TEAM CONFERENCE DECISIONS

Mary W., the utilization review coordinator, reviews Progress Notes within 24 to 48 hours of each team conference. For the first and second team conference on a patient, she simply checks to see that goals are identified and that there are statements about progress. Beginning with the third team conference, which occurs after two extended periods of stay, Mary reviews the team conference notes with a "physician advisor," who must be consulted for further assignment of days for continued stay. If the advisor agrees with the team's decision and recommendations, he authorizes them; if the advisor is not in agreement, both advisor and attending physician (the latter presides at the conference) attempt to work out their differences. If they cannot, the matter is brought to the attention of one of the two physician consultants who are staff physiatrists but who do not have direct responsibilities for individual patient care at the hospital, and they attempt to mediate the dispute. If they are still not able to resolve the matter, it may come before the hospital's utilization review committee where a final decision is reached. For the most part, disagreement over the results of team conferences is rare. When disagreements do occur, they are routinely resolved on the first level of the formal review apparatus.

According to Mary, the review following the first and second team conference has its typical problems, commonly omissions. Sometimes a physician forgets to specify the reason for continued hospitalization. She then approaches him or her and asks that the report be completed. On occasion a physician makes no specific recommendation, or the therapists' Notes do not clearly identify goals or progress. In those instances she asks for "clarification," which is a request that the Notes be revised or amended. She knows that two physicians are "particularly sloppy" in doing their Notes. Although they are both "good doctors," she looks at their Notes more carefully than the others.

In addition to problems created by omissions and careless entries, one is created by an older physician who Mary believes "does not like to discharge patients." This doctor has had a hard time adjusting to the "harsh realities" of utilization review and "cares only about patient needs, not about containing costs." The problem created by reluctance to discharge is compounded by the fact that Dr. P. also is an unreliable report writer. Mary is never sure whether "Dr. P forgot to record progress and goals or simply doesn't like to discharge the patient." Wilshire's response to this problem and to related physician idiosyncracies was to prepare a form letter which is sent to the patient and the family shortly before discharge. The letter explains that Medicare or Medicaid payment will terminate on a particular date. It states that an extension of up to three days may be granted if the patient experiences "difficulties in making arrangements for further care," but that the patient will probably be personally responsible for all bills and fees beyond the date specified. Staff consider the letter to be unduly harsh but necessary as a last resort in covering them in final discharge decisions.

Another problem arises from the interpersonal dislikes of certain physicians. When there is friction between a physician advisor and an attending physician and the justification for extended stay is not well documented, the advisor is less likely to approve routinely the decision or to work out an informal agreement to strengthen the justification. Mary once described a persistent antagonism between a male and a female physician. The female doctor had been assigned to cover some of his patients and to chair his team conferences while he was on vacation. In a couple of cases she failed to provide reason for continued hospitalization and the physician advisor on duty recommeded discharge. She agreed with his decision and praised the hospital's cost-containment efforts. However, when her own patients were at issue she apparently was not as agreeable. Mary noted that this male physician often served as a physician advisor and that he "got picky" whenever he reviewed his female colleague's recommendations for extended stays. He might not certify them or agree reluctantly but request further documentation. In one case he wrote the following message in the section of the review form reserved for comments on justifications for extended stay: "If team [conference] due 7/2/79 cannot demonstrate distinct gains, pt. should be discharged." When her patients were not certified for continued stay or when she received reviews like this one, this physician became extremely angry and claimed undue interference in medical discretion. According to Mary, after several similar reviews, the female physician became more circumspect in assessing what was submitted for the Team Conference Notes, prodding therapists to be more complete in their Progress Notes.

As review advisors the doctors vary in their dependability, in Mary's opinion. Some of them meet with her at scheduled times; others must be rounded up, even reminded that they are the advisor for the day. Whatever the effort involved in arranging reviews, Mary prepares to discuss the submitted Progress Notes. As she reviews them, she locates the ones that might pose problems in third-party claims reviews. As she presents the Notes and reports to the physician advisor, she guides the latter's considerations with comments such as "No problem with these" or "You might want to look at this one." When Mary recommends approval, the advisor normally glances at the Notes briefly and then signs the form authorizing, for example, an extended stay. If there is a problem, Mary points it out and they discuss what to do. Mary may volunteer to meet informally with the attending physician and/or therapists if it is unclear whether they are recommending continued stay or discharge, or if goals or progress are not adequately identified. Sometimes the advisor himself approaches the attending physician.

Regardless of the manner in which problems and disagreements surrounding hospitalization, continued rehab procedures, and discharge matters are resolved, their complications are not evident for the most part in what is made available to third parties. Team conference reviews are a final, formal assurance of this, the last link in a chain of descriptive practices that medically justify rehabilitative treatment.

Chapter 6

Accountability

To be accountable is to be subject to having to report, describe, explain, or justify. We all are accountable in one way or another in our everyday lives as we are called upon or feel the need to describe activities and events to a variety of others—family, friends, colleagues, clients, neighbors, subordinates, and superiors. In the process we take into consideration both accuracy and adequacy. We consider not only the truth of what we describe but the audience to whom we present it. We take for granted that proper/ acceptable descriptions are not simply valid depictions, but are worked up and offered in particular circumstances. To articulate descriptions in and with respect to situations and audiences is not principally a matter of deception, although deception may be a more or less accurate way to assess particular descriptions. Rather it is to be responsive to the practical matters of the descriptive process. To have available a description which can be judged for accuracy and/or acceptability, whether formally or informally, is first to produce it—something which is, while seemingly obvious, an integral but mostly tacit feature of concern over accountability.

There is another way of conceiving accountability, which is narrower, more formal, more restricted. In principle, its descriptive activity is thought to differ in quality from description in everyday life. Circumstance, interpretation, and audience do not intrude except as accountability is poorly or deceitfully done. It is chiefly a technical enterprise, one whose standards are the validity and reliability of description. Sometimes called "professional" or "scientific" accountability, its purpose is a special one—to demonstrate the effectiveness and efficiency of programs and applications.

In this chapter we examine the relationship between descriptive practice and accountability. The narrower, formal sense of the relationship is treated first. This is the perspective adopted by many policymakers, evaluators, applied social scientists, and human service workers. It is the perspective that frames evaluations of Wilshire staff members' descriptions of rehabilitation. Second, we turn to several views and issues concerning the limits and possibilities of accountability as formally conceived.

FORMAL ACCOUNTABILITY

The modern "accountability movement" may be traced to an increasing desire for public discourse in the wake of participating electorates as legitimate objects of governmental service (Gouldner, 1976) and to the rise of the welfare state (Greer, Hedlund, and Gibson, 1978). As public institutions and bureaucracies have taken over an increasing share of human services, once provided in other ways, and added new services, questions have naturally arisen about how well the public is being served—issues which are, rightly or wrongly, said to be difficult for the citizenry or their representatives to judge. Most bureaucracies are large, complex, and insulated from their clients and funding sources. Those who staff them speak a strange, professional language. While professionals claim to be working in the public interest, can this be concretely shown?

There are at least three general strategies for answering the question. One locates solutions in conditions external to professional human service activity and description. A popular variety is to recommend more competition and consumer choice. We might have a voucher system in education or alternatives to the health care systems currently controlled by the medical establishment. The worth of these competing services, that is, their quality and cost, may then be appraised in much the same way as those offered by private enterprises operating in a competitive market economy. Efficient and effective institutions are those that survive or prosper at the expense of others. Another solution is to encourage alternate patterns of governance by means of decentralization and the provision of greater access to judicial review and relief (Lipsky, 1978).

A second strategy offers a bureaucratic approach to what is seen as essentially a bureaucratic problem. Greater accountability lies in making human service bureaucracies what they should be ideally: highly rational organizations. Part of the solution depends on recruiting employees with better training and in selecting people who are professionally certified for the work. There is also a need for increased rationalization of the relationship between process and outcome. Organizational activity should be made more explicit, objectified in quantitative terms. This strategy is represented in such well-known management and accounting schemes as zero-based budgeting, program planning budgeting systems, cost-benefit analysis, and management by objective (Miringoff, 1980). Accountability is achieved through better administrative control (Lipsky, 1978).

A third strategy allies the administrative with the social sciences in the pursuit of accountability. Internal controls, such as those identified under the second strategy, allow human service institutions to be more precise in describing process and goals. They can specify eligibility requirements, clarify rationales which link services with problems, and demonstrate benefits and costs. An external agent also becomes involved, when reports on the internal monitoring of management and service provision are required for review. External reviewers may also be given another, perhaps more important, responsibility: evaluating outcomes. Outcome evaluation goes beyond checking the efficiency of management to measuring program effectiveness. The significant question becomes: Do the services provided make some difference in select areas of the lives of clients, when judged against a relevant baseline or comparative measure? Or does one service approach demonstrate superiority over another in this regard? (Nachmias, 1978; Rossi and Williams, 1972; Weiss, 1972). Judgments of either inefficiency or ineffectiveness might lead to denial of payment for services rendered, reductions in or withholding of future funding, or similar sanctions.

The PSRO is an example of the third strategy. Individual hospitals are held responsible for formalizing their internal clinical management. They are required to establish administrative policies, following local or regional guidelines, and carefully monitor decision-making in such matters as admissions, length of hospitalization, and quality and appropriateness of treatment. Problems are identified through claims reviews and the analysis of case data in "medical care evaluation studies." Using data provided by individual hospitals, the PSRO monitors performance in each, through the review of all or a sample of cases, and conducts studies of the cost and quality of treatment on a regional basis (Chassin, 1978; Goran, 1979).

DISSENTING VIEWS

While it is unfashionable to be against accountability in principle, a variety of issues have been raised which, in one way or another, point to aspects which make it more or less than simply a matter of objective, valid, or reliable reporting, evaluation, and decision-making.

Politics and Accountability

Etzioni (1975) provides perhaps the most general critique of professional accountability envisioned as a scientifically valid and reliable system of description and method for rational assessment and control. He points out that there are alternative conceptions of, and several other functions for, accountability schemes. In suggesting that accountability is a political symbol, he points to how appeals for, or claims of, accountability are used to rally persons behind a cause or to assuage critics with promises of improved performance. Accountability also serves *"realpolitik"*; powerbrokers manipulate the rules of the game so that accountability feeds their interests and purposes.

Etzioni distinguishes a "formal" and "guidance" model of accountability. The PSRO is an organization conceived in terms of the formal model, where professionals are held to rules, laws, and procedures. While Etzioni holds that this model produces some positive effects, he argues that informal networks and tacit conspiracies compromise the purity of the design. He prefers the latter, the guidance model, which combines the rules and procedures of the formal approach with the active, creative participation of professional staff and administrators in adopting operating procedures and reporting practices to satisfy a variety of changing situations and power relationships. In Etzioni's view, professionals can be accountable, but they should not be locked into a formal, rigid system that prevents creative flexibility and maneuvering. An effective system of accountability must allow for changing political relationships and coalitions and the identification of and response to new alternatives.

Service Interests

A critique of "scientific" accountability questions whether the evaluation of descriptive accounts of service activities can be separated from varying service interests. The goals and procedures of any human service institution cannot be evaluated apart from a consideration of whom it serves. For example, Wynne (1976) argues that public schools might be accountable to a variety of groups, including taxpayers, educational experts, and parents. Each group is likely to have a somewhat different view of what should be happening in schools and demand what may be conflicting goals for and information about process and outcome. Wynne's own choice of parents as the proper audience and an educational system focused on character development, moral soundness, and good work habits would most likely make for a different style and substance of reporting about schooling than would a system of accountability addressed to another audience.

The issue of service interest is also raised by some who question the ability of professionals to control and regulate themselves. Self-regulation is an important feature of professional socialization and identification but it has come under criticism in recent years, both as a general issue and as a concern with the behavior of specific professional groups like physicians (Freidson, 1973). Freidson and Rhea (1965), for example, argue that while, as a group, physicians claim that only they can regulate one another's professional behavior, in practice they are reluctant to intervene in each other's business—to do so is considered unprofessional. The creation of an administrative structure, such as the PSRO, to oversee and promote accountable behavior is not without problems of its own. Freidson (1976) notes that physicians are far from passive participants in the utilization review process, and that, depending on their interest, they will attempt to manipulate the monitoring apparatus to suit their own ends. Cohen (1975) discusses the "capture theory" of regulatory agencies and applies it to the operation of the PSRO, where select physicians are responsible for overseeing the practices of other physicians. He argues that substantive rather than procedural regulation should be the major concern, even though the latter is likely to receive most attention. As a result, doctors may alter their reporting practices but not their behavior. One implication seems to be that with a different membership, with different service interests, the PSRO would be able to effect both substantive and procedural accountability. Cohen points out that physicians themselves do not have homogeneous service interests, such as varying commitments to group versus solo practice or fee versus prepaid service. These add an internal component to the variation in service interest that complicates accountability.

Greer (1978) traces the rationale for the PSRO to several conditions that have eroded confidence in scientific medicine. These include increasing costs, medicine's poor scientific status and the outdated knowledge of many doctors, and the recognition that better food, sanitation, and disease prevention are more important to health than medical care. The desire for regulation, however, has been complicated by differing perspectives and interests: national and local, public and private, professional and lay. Cutting accross these are the "professional monopolists" and the "bureaucratic rationalizers" (Alford, 1976). The monopolists are those who aim to protect their current interests in a winning game while the rationalizers seek more control and bureaucratic predictability. In comparison, organized consumers, as an interest group, have little political clout. The PSRO is a political compromise between the two interests with power. It is a conservative solution in terms of consumers and may result in what Greer describes, again following Alford, as "dynamics without change." To avoid this and to provide for a better outcome for all concerned parties, Greer suggests an additional layer of accountability: a review of the reviewers. The mechanisms for this would be drawn from the research tools of social science, their operation presumably being entrusted to neutral social scientists.

Unintended Consequences

The common view of accountability portrays it as either an additive component of bureaucratic structure, a reporting and evaluative element, or as a positive interactive component—one which shapes or constrains other elements in a desirable, rational way. It tends to gloss over the possibility of unintended and often undesirable effects when performance is formally held accountable, particularly by means of quantitative measures.

The classic statement of this problem is found in Blau's study (1963) of employment counselors who began focusing their efforts on easy-to-place clients at the expense of more difficult cases once the criterion for assessing their work was shifted from handling caseloads to successful placements. Lipsky (1980) describes a number of similar examples of unintended consequences. Social workers may "cream" when they recruit clients for their programs: they select only those likely to do well in order to enhance their image of success. While the police claim a large reduction in the rate of serious crime, they fail to report an increase in the number of burglaries involving items with an estimated value of under $50, which is the cutoff point for defining a burglary as serious. Teachers focus their instruction on what they know will be tested at the expense of what they see as more important educational objectives.

Lipsky rejects the argument that unintended and unwanted consequences are due simply to badly trained, poorly motivated employees, or lax management. Instead he traces the difficulty to the extremely complex job of what he labels "street-level bureaucrats" —human service workers who work on a face-to-face basis with individual clients. These include teachers, social workers, probation officers, the police, and health care professionals. The work of street-level bureaucrats requires considerable discretion in responding to the needs of individual clients in ways that are also feasible and proper within the bureaucracy. Formal rules or guidelines do not adequately spell out proper procedure in individual cases. Workers must formulate creative, discretionary solutions within the limits placed on them by the bureaucracy. But quantitative measures of performance, which are used for comparative and evaluative purposes, assume standard practices with known outcomes and some degree of control over the difficulty and complexity of client problems. Lipsky argues that these assumptions do not hold and that we both fail to appreciate the complexity of human service work and force street-level bureaucrats to change their behavior in undesirable ways when we attempt to judge the quality of work through quantitative accounting.

Hoshino (1973) has similar concerns. He cites many of the same problems identified by Lipsky and adds that the substitution of quantitative reports of work performance for the conventional narrative summary may lead to two undesirable outcomes for workers and clients: human service workers who, on the one hand, learn to fill out forms to show desired results without changing their behavior or those, on the other hand, who tighten their control on client behavior with more regard to work rules or procedure than the needs of the clients.

Weinbach (1977) also identifies unintended consequences, but his concern is more with the public status of human service workers than with the problem of reporting. Focusing on social work, he argues that the rewards of money and prestige have lured social workers into claiming professional status. What they do not realize, or choose to overlook, he maintains, is that professionalism assumes clear goals, a scientific base, and cause-effect relationships between services offered and outcomes achieved. The inevitable result of a claim of professional status is a demand for accountability, a demand which cannot be met. Social workers cannot demonstrate either efficiency or instrumentality. Even if outcomes could be measured, they are unable to show the cost-effectiveness of their services or a necessary relationship between services and outcomes. Weinbach recommends that social workers attempt to escape the shackles of accountability by lowering their professional sights and insisting on a comparative judgement with their competitors—psychologists and psychiatrists. He obviously feels that the competitors are in no better position to support a claim of professional status.

Freidson (1975, 1976) warns that there are real dangers when those concerned rely on formal modes of administrative measurement and reporting for their data. The façade of accountability may conceal important qualitative aspects of service provision. While Freidson dwells on health care, Douglas (1971) discusses the problem as it applies to a broad range of human service work. They both warn that an increasing reliance on external and technical reporting for knowledge of social processes and outcomes are blinding us to the rich detail and dynamics of social life. Theory, and thus understanding, are bound to suffer.

Record Production

The work of Freidson and Douglas might also be included within another perspective which in part raises questions about the objective status of bureaucratic records. It is based on studies of the social processes through which record-making is managed or accomplished in bureaucratic settings. While there is polemical undertone in some of this work, it is characterized less by direct attack on the scientific adequacy of formal accountability than by a theoretical commitment to study the social process and uses of administrative accounting without a prior commitment to some ideal model or to the special status of formal accountability as a highly rational, objective form of description. What is revealed is the practice of formal accounting.

Wheeler (1969), for example, calls for studies of the social processes through which organizational records are made, kept, and used for purposes of accountability. He argues that formal descriptions in bureaucratic settings are constructed by describers who have their own purposes and concerns and are not simply passive, objective reflectors of client and staff behavior. Both what is contained in records and how the records are read are articulated through values, biases, and interests. In short, description is *done*, by and for someone, under certain conditions. Much of this is concealed by official rhetoric, which principally presents records as only about the reality of clients. This stance has advantages for official users. It creates the appearance of legitimacy and objectivity, allows for the combination of isolated aspects of a case into a coherent story, and facilitates interorganizational communication and division of labor. Wheeler exhorts social scientists to see through the official rhetoric and to conduct studies which will contribute to a better understanding of the social dynamics of record production.

Studies of the social organization of record production have been undertaken by a number of investigators. Lemert (1969) discusses the production and use of files in the juvenile court. He finds no clear professional logic to what information is included in a file and what is omitted and little correspondence between the contents of records and recommendations for action. A variety of implicit factors may influence what goes into a record, from the demeanor of the child to the social class of the family. A judge can usually find a rationale in the record for his decision even though the most important factors have nothing to do with a particular case. For example, community pressure to get tough on juveniles may overshadow the facts on record. The situation is made more complex by the realization that "reasonable" facts may be retroactively added to support a decision or that probation officers and others may select certain facts or push certain interpretations in their courtroom presentations in order to influence a judge's decision by, say, playing on his "pet peeves."

Erikson and Gilbertson (1969) discuss the production and use of records in mental hospitals. They argue that files are read as containing flat, static, one-dimensional facts when in reality the construction process is highly textured by circumstance. They are written for and by physicians in the language they prefer while other ways of reporting, and other facts, are never recorded. Files contain a kind of folklore. They are assembled in order to demonstrate sickness and to make commitment reasonable. They also serve to justify particular forms of treatment and to document change.

Public welfare agencies have also been sites for studies of record production (Zimmerman, 1969). Administrative records have several uses. They establish the eligibility of clients for the services offered by the agency. They also certify whatever actions are taken on their behalf and establish factual descriptions of the organization's related conduct. Most documents are taken for granted to be authentic, valid traces of a principally ordered and rational world. The world of the client is taken for granted to stand independent of its documentation by staff; it is described by "plain facts." When for some reason or other a record becomes problematic, staff artfully work to develop a clear interpretation, often involving new facts, which makes a decision warrantable. Such practical solutions sustain the image of an orderly bureaucratic process over the vagaries of everyday practical contingencies.

Other studies which at least in part examine the practical grounds from which ostensibly objective records are produced and used for purposes of accountability include Cicourel (1968), Leiter (1974), Gubrium and Buckholdt (1977, 1979), Buckholdt and Gubrium (1979a, b, 1980), and Gubrium (1980a). The organizations studied range from the juvenile court to the public school, the residential treatment center, and the nursing home. The variety supports the generality of record production in the accountability of service organizations.

Following theoretical leads of Goffman (1959) and Lyman and Scott (1970), Altheide and Johnson (1980) argue for the relevance of a dramaturgical perspective in understanding organizational reporting or, as they call it, "bureaucratic propaganda." The work that goes into the presentation of an organizational self supplies the topic for their investigation. They consider the place of "image" and "audience" in the construction of bureaucratic reports. While the reality of events, accomplishments, or behavior is officially at issue, behind the scenes they find practical concerns for legitimacy defined in terms of qualities such as efficiency, objectivity, and rationality. Reports are prepared and edited with particular audiences in mind and the descriptions that emerge are products of "anticipation-inspired performances"—clever activities said to be organizationally and professionally self-serving. Altheide's and Johnson's aim is both to document the artificial underside of bureaucratic propaganda and to provide their readers with an awareness of the gap between appearance and reality.

One of the bureaucratic settings described by Altheide and Johnson was a public welfare agency. In addition to preparing routine written narratives on their contacts with clients, welfare workers were periodically asked to provide quantitative data on such matters as the number and types of clients they contacted and how they distributed their time among different types of clients. The authors describe several practical considerations not revealed in the counts that emerged. For example, individual workers worried about, and sometimes adjusted their counts in consideration of, how their own numbers would compare with those of colleagues, and how the differences would be evaluated and perhaps used against them. Members of a unit debated how to assemble a report, given their desire to have more caseworkers or to avoid cutbacks in funding. Together with other practical concerns, these led to strategies for reporting that included the consideration of audience expectations and intended effects. It was obvious that similar concerns were also operating at higher levels of the bureaucracy, for reports were sometimes "kicked back" several times until they revealed what administrators wanted them to show.

ACCOUNTING PRACTICE

Descriptive work involves describers in the practical process of considering the truth about what is described as well as the adequacy of those descriptions. This holds whether description is casual, as, for example, that frequently offered to patients or family members, or formal, such as when patient progress is reported to outside agencies. Matters of practice and adequacy present a persistent problem for formal models of accountability. Formal models assume that accountability can be judged principally on grounds of accuracy and consistency. But there is a broader relationship between description and accountability, one informed by this and other studies of descriptive practice.

In the broader view, professional accountability is seen as a variety of "accounting practice." (See Mehan and Wood, 1975, and Leiter, 1980, for a review of the literature.) Accounting practices are not technical devices. They are reality-defining and reality-sustaining methods whereby objects of concern are both reported on and made observable—that is, real and objective. From this point of view, what we have reported in the preceding chapters describes the accounting practices of a group of professionals at work in a rehabilitation hospital. The content of their descriptions is of interest in that it defines the objects and events that are real to them—the possible images of the way things are in physical rehabilitation. Also important for our purposes, however, are the social processes through which reality is constructed for particular audiences.

Is there a way to produce valid and accurate reports without image and audience effects, without interpretive discretion? Can we divorce ourselves from the descriptive process and report only on what is "really and truly" there as objective fact? This, of course, is the goal of much professional concern with description. That professionals are aware of problems in implementing such an ideal is recognized in dealing with troublesome conditions such as bias, invalidity, unreliability, and measurement error. It is, understood, however, that these conditions can be overcome through better training, scientific controls, stricter documentation requirements, and similar solutions.

Critics of current forms of accountability and the descriptive activity on which they depend generally remain sanguine about the future of objective reporting and rational decision-making and control. Their optimism is bolstered by a variety of arguments. One is based on studies which show that some institutions or professionals behave in a more responsible manner than others. The claim that some are doing better than others provides for the possibility of overall improvement. For example, studies of hospital utilization and medical treatment, by region, show wide variations on such measures as average length of stay for selected diagnoses and the likelihood of hospitalization given certain ailments (Goran, 1979). One possible implication is that some PSROs and review structures are functioning better than others. Other evidence comes from research which shows large differences in the quality of record-keeping among different types of medical institutions. For example, where there is normative preference for patient care as opposed to teaching-research duties, the former reduces the quality of medical records (Nathanson and Becker, 1973). Indeed, it has been suggested that the quality of care can be judged from the quality of record-keeping (Donabedian, 1969). Another argument rests on the promises of evaluation research methodology. With the advent of more sophisticated statistical techniques and research designs, we should be able to sort out truthful claims about matters like rehabilitation from false ones (Nachmias 1978). And finally, there is the hope offered by new modes of information processing. Lemert (1969), for example, foresees the day when automated data systems will make courts, police, and probation officers more accountable to their clients and the public by rapidly and concisely revealing inefficiency, bias, and lack of due process. He does not explain, however, how the discretionary practices he discusses in current forms of reading and reporting will be eliminated by computers.

Wilshire staff members share in this optimism. While they recognize and on occasion openly discuss how their descriptive

practices are influenced by situational and audience considerations, the recognition is well contained and does not threaten their
confidence in their ability to report the truth of clinical matters.
For example, a PT explained to a social worker that optimistic
statements about progress were exaggerated in a particular case
in order to spark the motivation of a patient and his wife. Similar
assessments made in a Progress Note were intended to convince
the PSRO that further hospitalization was justified and indeed the
PT thought it was, but more because the therapist believed the
patient's potential to be more than actual progress to date. The
therapist made it clear, however, that if the physician were to ask
her about the patient's real status, only minimal gain would be
reported. The difference was considered to be a matter of being
practical. If called upon to provide an objective account, stripped
of all practical concerns, like others, the therapist believes this
could be accomplished. A physician expressed a similar understanding of descriptive variation when discussing the importance
of the utilization review during a team conference:

> I know some of you wanted to discharge Mrs. Marty, but we can't
> just yet. There still are some things we can do for her and, besides,
> her family isn't ready for her just now. Be a little patient, she won't
> be with us much longer. I think we're getting better at pinpointing
> problems, you know, really being able to measure them. Sometime
> down the pike this will be pretty much a really straightforward
> process. We won't have to change our story to catch up with what's
> happening. Mind you, I'm not criticizing the way we do things, but
> I am sure, down the pike, we'll have more scientific ways to quantify
> our work. We should begin now to pay more attention to evidence.
> When you make an assessment of a patient, always include the
> evidence to back it up and try to report objective evidence, like counts
> of things or how long they were able to do something.

"Descriptive practice" differs from the "bureaucratic propaganda" discussed by Altheide and Johnson (1980). Implied in the
latter is a belief in the possibility of practice-free, audience-free
accounts, the possibility of "nonpropagandistic" description—
something that informs the optimism of both critics of accountability and its practitioners. Altheide and Johnson argue that
truth in bureaucratic reporting has a practical context that involves the consideration of what is needed to achieve various goals.
Reports have a career, a purpose, and a meaning in their own right
and are not just better or worse reflections of some reality. Our
analysis is like theirs to this point. However, they make a theo-

retical, not an empirically problematic, distinction between "appearance" and "reality," and here we differ. Their distinction suggests the possibility of obtaining a descriptive semblance of reality unencumbered by practice and its concrete considerations. Thus one might be able to see beyond bureaucratic propaganda to what is really happening. While another reality could be portrayed, its descriptive activity also would involve purposes, contexts, and considerations of adequacy. It is impossible, in our view, to achieve a method of reporting devoid of practice. Whether known or unknown, description is always done by someone, within the confines of purposes and duties at hand, and more or less wittingly stands to be offered to someone else. It becomes propaganda only in its presentation or acceptance as such. The distinction between appearance and reality is an ongoing problem for those concerned with it (all of us), not a standard against which we can objectively judge others for substance and rhetoric.

To speak of descriptive practice is to delimit accountability. It is to recognize something that is an obvious, but for that reason, usually hidden feature of speaking, informing, and reporting. Describers, audiences, circumstance, and image are part and parcel of the accomplishment of description. These are the limits of accountability. The acceptability of accounts cannot be separated from them.

Thus, in considering what clinical staff at Wilshire variously describe as rehabilitation, we encounter the inherent "contradictions" of everyday life in and about the institution, "contradictions" that, in practice, organize what is descriptively reasonable about treatment and care. While political, technical, and administrative solutions to "problems" of accountability might affect the style and content of description, they can not eclipse its practical considerations.

References

Alford, Robert. 1976. *Health Care Politics: Ideological and Interest Group Barriers to Reform.* Chicago: University of Chicago Press.

Altheide, David L., and John M. Johnson. 1980. *Bureaucratic Propaganda.* Boston: Allyn and Bacon.

Berger, Peter, and Thomas Luckmann. 1966. *The Social Construction of Reality.* New York: Doubleday.

Blau, Peter M. 1963. *The Dynamics of Bureaucracy.* Chicago: University of Chicago Press.

Buckholdt, David R., and Jaber F. Gubrium. 1979a. *Caretakers: Treating Emotionally Disturbed Children.* Beverly Hills, Calif.: Sage.

———. 1979b. "Doing Staffings." *Human Organization,* 38:255–264.

———. 1980. "The Underlife of Behavior Modification." *American Journal of Orthopsychiatry,* 50:279–290.

Chassin, Mark R. 1978. "The Containment of Hospital Costs: A Strategic Assessment." *Medical Care,* 10:1–55.

Cicourel, Aaron V. 1968. *The Social Organization of Juvenile Justice.* New York: Wiley.

Cicourel, Aaron V. et al. 1974. *Language Use and School Performance.* New York: Academic Press.

Cicourel, Aaron V., and John I. Kitsuse. 1963. *The Educational Decision Makers.* Indianapolis: Bobbs-Merrill.

Cohen, Harry. 1975. "Regulatory Politics and American Medicine." *American Behavioral Scientist,* 19:122–136.

Donabedian, Avedis. 1969. *Medical Care Appraisal: Quality and Utiliza-*

tion. *A Guide to Medical Care Administration,* Vol. 2. New York: Public Health Administration.

Douglas, Jack D. 1971. *American Social Order.* New York: Free Press.

Erikson, Kai T., and Daniel E. Gilbertson. 1969. "Case Records in the Mental Hospital." Pp. 389–412 in Stanton Wheeler (ed.), *On Record: Files and Dossiers in American Life.* New York: Russell Sage.

Etzioni, Amitai. 1975. "Alternative Conceptions of Accountability: The Example of Health Administration." *Public Administration Review,* 3:279–286.

Freidson, Eliot. 1975. *Doctoring Together: A Study of Professional Social Control.* New York: Elsevier.

———. 1976. "The Development of Administrative Accountability in Health Services." *American Behavioral Scientist,* 19:286–298.

Freidson, Eliot (ed.). 1973. *The Professions and their Prospects.* Beverly Hills, Calif.: Sage.

Freidson, Eliot and Buford Rhea. 1965. "Knowledge and Judgment in Professional Evaluations." *Administrative Science Quarterly,* 10:107–124.

Garfinkel, Harold. 1967. *Studies in Ethnomethodology.* Englewood Cliffs, N.J.: Prentice-Hall.

Glaser, Barney G. and Anselm L. Strauss. 1965. *Awareness of Dying.* Chicago: Aldine.

Goffman, Erving. 1959. *The Presentation of Self in Everyday Life.* Garden City, New York: Doubleday.

———. 1974. *Frame Analysis.* New York: Harper.

Goran, Michael J. 1979. "The Evolution of the PSRO Hospital Review System." *Medical Care,* 17:1–47.

Gouldner, Alvin W. 1976. *The Dialectic of Ideology and Technology.* New York: Seabury.

Greer, Scott. 1978. "Professional Self Regulation in the Public Interest: The Intellectual Politics of PSRO." Pp. 39–60 in Scott Greer, Ronald D. Hedlund and James L. Gibson (eds.), *Accountability in Urban Society.* Beverly Hills, Calif.: Sage.

Greer, Scott, Ronald D. Hedlund, and James L. Gibson. 1978. "Introduction: The Accountability of Institutions in Urban Society." Pp. 9-12 in Scott Greer, Ronald D. Hedlund, and James L. Gibson (eds.), *Accountability in Urban Society.* Beverly Hills, Calif.: Sage.

Gubrium, Jaber F. 1980a. "Doing Care Plans in Patient Conferences." *Social Science and Medicine,* 14A:659–667.

———. 1980b. "Patient Exclusion in Geriatric Staffings." *Sociological Quarterly,* 21:335–347.

Gubrium, Jaber F. and David R. Buckholdt. 1977. *Toward Maturity: The Social Processing of Human Development.* San Francisco: Jossey-Bass.

———. 1979. "Production of Hard Data in Human Service Institutions." *Pacific Sociological Review,* 22:115–136.

Gutmann, David. 1964. "An Exploration of Ego Configurations in Middle and Later Life." Pp. 114–148 in Bernice Neugarten (ed.), *Personality in Middle and Later Life.* New York: Atherton.

———. 1969. "The Country of Old Men: Cross-cultural Studies in the Psychology of Later Life." In W. Donahue (ed.), *Occasional Papers in Gerontology.* Ann Arbor: Institute of Gerontology, University of Michigan.

Hoshino, George. 1973. "Social Services: The Problem of Accountability." *The Social Services Review,* 47:373–383.

Krohn, A. and David Gutmann. 1971. "Changes in Mastery Style with Age: A Study of Navajo Dreams." *Psychiatry,* 34:289–300.

Leiter, Kenneth C.W. 1974. "Adhocing in the Schools: A Study of Placement Practices in the Kindergartens of Two Schools." Pp. 17–75 in Aaron Cicourel, et al., *Language Use and School Performance.* New York: Academic Press.

———. 1980. *A Primer on Ethnomethodology.* New York: Oxford University Press.

Lemert, Edwin M. 1969. "Records in the Juvenile Court." Pp. 355–387 in Stanton Wheeler (ed.), *On Record: Files and Dossiers in American Life.* New York: Russell Sage.

Lipsky, Michael. 1978. "The Assault on Human Services: Street-Level Bureaucrats, Accountability and the Fiscal Crisis." Pp. 15–38 in Scott Greer, Ronald D. Hedlund, and James L. Gibson (eds.), *Accountability in Urban Society.* Beverly Hills, Calif.: Sage.

———1980. *Street-Level Bureaucracy: Dilemmas of the Individual in Public Services.* New York: Russell Sage.

Lyman, Stanford M. and Marvin B. Scott. 1970. *The Sociology of the Absurd.* New York: Appleton-Century-Crofts.

Mehan, Hugh B. and H. Laurence Wood. 1975. *The Reality of Ethnomethodology.* New York: Wiley.

Miringoff, Marc L. 1980. *Management in Human Service Organizations.* New York: Macmillan.

Nachmias, David. 1978. *Public Policy Evaluation.* New York: St. Martin's Press.

Nathanson, Constance A. and Marshall Becker. 1973. "Doctors, Nurses, and Clinical Records." *Medical Care,* 11:214–223.

Rossi, Peter H. and Walter Williams (eds.). 1972. *Evaluating Social Programs: Theory, Practice, and Politics.* New York: Academic Press.

Schutz, Alfred. 1962. "On Multiple Realities." Pp. 207–259 in *Collected Papers I: The Problem of Social Reality.* Ed. by Maurice Natansen. The Hague: Nijhoff.

Weinbach, Robert W. 1977. "Accountability Crises: Consequences of Professionalization." *Journal of Sociology and Social Welfare,* 14:1011–1024.

Weiss, Carol H. (ed.) 1972. *Evaluating Action Programs: Readings in Social Action and Education.* Boston: Allyn and Bacon.

Wheeler, Stanton (ed.). 1969. *On Record: Files and Dossiers in American Life.* New York: Russell Sage.

Wynne, Edward. 1976. "Accountable to Whom." *Society,* 13:30–37.

Zimmerman, Don H. 1969. "Record-Keeping and the Intake Process in a Public Welfare Agency." Pp. 319–354 in Stanton Wheeler (ed.), *On*

Record: Files and Dossiers in American Life. New York: Russell Sage.

Zimmerman, Don H., and Melvin Pollner. 1970. "The Everyday World as a Phenomenon." Pp. 80–103 in Jack Douglas (ed.), *Understanding Everyday Life.* Chicago: Aldine.

Index

191

About the Authors

Jaber F. Gubrium is Professor of Sociology at Marquette University and Director of its program on Aging and the Life Cycle. He has been interested in the social organization of care and treatment in human service institutions and, most currently, in the descriptive activity of service providers. Dr. Gubrium is the author of *Living and Dying at Murray Manor*, an ethnography of the differential worlds of care in a nursing home. He recently completed *Toward Maturity: The Social Processing of Human Development* and *Caretakers* with David Buckholdt.

David R. Buckholdt is Associate Professor and Chairman of the Department of Sociology and Anthropology at Marquette University. His first book, *The Humanization Processes* (with Robert Hamblin and others) reports research on instructional and curricular innovation in public schools. Since joining the Marquette faculty in 1974, Dr. Buckholdt has concerned himself with the development of a social interactional approach to human development and the study of decision making and descriptive activity in human service institutions. His books *Toward Maturity: The Social Processing of Human Development* and *Caretakers* (with Jaber Gubrium) reflect the more recent interests.